PERFECTING THE PIG ENVIRONMENT

P Smith

Pork Chain Solutions Ltd and PIGSPEC

N Bird

Farmex Ltd

HG Crabtree

Farmex Ltd

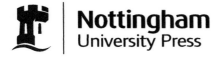
Nottingham
University Press

Nottingham University Press
Manor Farm, Main Street, Thrumpton
Nottingham, NG11 0AX, United Kingdom
www.nup.com

NOTTINGHAM

First published 2009
© P. Smith, N. Bird and H.G. Crabtree

British Library Cataloguing in Publication Data
Perfecting the Pig Environment

ISBN 978-1904761-81-5

Disclaimer

Every reasonable effort has been made to ensure that the material in this book is true, correct, complete and appropriate at the time of writing. Nevertheless the publishers, the editors and the authors do not accept responsibility for any omission or error, or for any injury, damage, loss or financial consequences arising from the use of the book.

Typeset by Nottingham University Press, Nottingham
Printed and bound by MPG Books Group in the UK

CONTENTS

Preface   v

Introduction   vii

1   Environmental monitoring – theory, common practice and   1
best practice.

2   The impact of stocking density – pigs generates heat and   11
increasingly need space.

3   Data interpretation – making the most of environmental   15
monitoring.

4   Temperature monitoring – a good starting point for   19
fine-tuning the pig environment.

5   Ventilation – the ultimate practical compromise.   29

6   Feed and water – always needed but rarely measured.   43

7   The consequences of excessive temperature build-up.   59

8   I.T. – the global driver of future pig production.   73

Index   83

Dedication

To those who keep pigs well and continuously strive to keep them better.

Acknowledgements

The authors are pleased to acknowledge the help of early-adopter pig farmers for their enthusiasm and willingness to co-operate and explore new technical opportunities. Thanks are due to a wide range of individuals and organisations involved in the diverse global pig industry and I.T. specialists from other industries. Help from Beverley Goldthorpe for her meticulous typing is gratefully acknowledged.

Preface

Like its predecessor, this publication is written for students and those professionals who choose to work at the 'sharp end' of the pig industry and are driven by a desire to improve the environment that farmers provide for pigs. The authors describe proven monitoring techniques which can also interpret data and automatically implement adjustments to environment control systems. Readers are led through a series of case studies from commercial pig farms. Explanations of the source of problems within pig buildings are provided and augmented by graphical data which are explained in simple terms. In particular, the book makes much reference to I.T. devices already in use within other industries and speculates how these will be increasingly used to help pig farmers integrate more closely with their food chain partners.

The authors, although academically trained, have years of experience communicating directly with pig farmers and those in allied industries. Paul Smith undertook applied research on pigs at the Agricultural Development and Advisory Service's Great House Experimental Husbandry Farm. He subsequently worked as ADAS Pig Specialist for Norfolk & East Suffolk and in 1987 created PIGSPEC, an independent consultancy operating in the private sector. He writes regularly in the technical farming press and in 2002 became a founder director of Pork Chain Solutions Ltd, an alliance of independent pig consultants. Nick Bird has had a major impact on the development of real time monitoring of the environment within pig and poultry buildings particularly within the United Kingdom and the United States of America. All the examples used in this publication have arisen from his on-farm case study work involving challenging problems on commercial farms. Both Nick Bird and Hugh Crabtree studied and then undertook postgraduate research in the Engineering Section of the Agriculture Department at Reading University. They were co-founders of Farm Energy & Control Systems Ltd in 1979 and since then have gained much practical experience assessing pig production efficiency in a range of environments. In 2006 Hugh Crabtree presented a paper entitled 'Can the Promise of IT become a Reality in Pig Production?' when he was the recipient of The Royal Agricultural College and National Westminster Bank 100 Club Annual Fellowship in Pig Research.

INTRODUCTION

In an earlier publication entitled "Pig Environment Problems" (ISBN 978-1-897676-18-9), an attempt was made to unveil the science of pig environment and to present it in a reader-friendly form. It was aimed at students, pig farmers and those working in allied industries. The increasing need for an ethical approach to pig production was emphasised along with social factors involving both farm worker and consumer issues. The broader aspects of the impact that pig keeping has on the environment beyond the farm were also discussed in some detail. The theory of thermal comfort, air movement principles and the impact of noxious gases on pigs and people were also considered. Theory is nothing more than a formal description of what happens in practice and must not be regarded as daunting by those with a natural affinity with the species. Such people tend to have a gift for understanding pigs and their environmental needs.

This follow-up publication assumes a basic knowledge of both the theory and practice of pig environment and confronts the challenge of getting it right and the expensive consequences of getting it wrong. The basic philosophy of the book is that 'You can't control what you don't measure.' It aims to demonstrate how systematic monitoring can expose shortcomings within the pig environment, their impact on profitability and suggests cost-effective ways of improving any unacceptable situation uncovered. The case studies presented are taken from commercial pig farms experiencing difficulties in providing the optimum environmental conditions. Environmental inadequacies can arise because of fundamental design faults in buildings and environment control systems. A lack of understanding of the biology and behaviour patterns of the pig might be the source of such problems. They might have arisen because insufficient attention was paid to commissioning a new installation; equipment failure could be another cause as could wear and tear over the years, possibly accelerated because of the absence of a regular maintenance plan. Furthermore, sometimes pigs fail to thrive in what seems to be the ideal environment; this could arise because clinically or sub clinically diseased pigs have been housed within it. Hence, an ability to confirm normality or recognise abnormality and implement remedial action are key elements in ensuring that pigs thrive within the optimum environment. It all gets back to regular monitoring.

The existence of a sub-standard pig environment reduces staff morale and commitment which impacts on pig health and profitability. Together, labour and feed represent well over 80 per cent of production costs; hence it is vital that a pig environment is provided which facilitates the efficient production of lean meat.

Ensuring that the pig is given the very best opportunity within the environment imposed on it demands a multi-disciplinary approach. Many parties are involved ranging from building manufacturers, building assemblers, equipment manufacturers and installation electricians as well as pig farmers and those who actually manage pig buildings. Despite research efforts providing the pig industry with crucial fundamental information, inadequate pig environments are both commonplace and costly. Pig farmers often have a range of enterprises and associated responsibilities and so demand sophistication and simplicity at the same time. How these systems are actually managed is the key issue.

Troubleshooting visits to problem pig environments regularly indicate shortcomings in the basics. Inadequacy in air inlet design is commonplace as is under-ventilation. The latter arises increasingly on pig units which have shifted from continuous throughput production to all-in/all-out systems often combined with higher slaughter weights. Other common problems are the existence of draughts at pig level, cold or wet lying areas and problems arising because of inappropriate stocking densities. Sometimes, there is a breakdown in the communication circle resulting in the person actually managing the pigs not being adequately briefed on the limitations of the control system.

How can a progressive pig industry address these issues? Pig environment and ventilation in particular must not become an afterthought when a new pig building is planned. The design and thinking process should be initiated at the earliest opportunity and should involve those who will manage the building. The responsibilities of those entrusted with the daily care of the pigs should be clearly defined and, where necessary, reputable specialist advice should be sought. This, very likely, would involve genetics, nutrition, pig welfare, pig health, farm waste and market outlet. When existing buildings are refurbished, on-gong problems must be clearly pinpointed and quantified, management practices reviewed and the need for any changes discussed in detail before implementation. This must be regarded as an integral part of any de-population and re-stocking strategy.

Getting the pig environment right is not easy, neither is it rocket science; it depends on an understanding of the basic principles involved. An appreciation of the need for steady state heat balance within the pig building and how the movement of air impacts on room temperature are crucial. All those involved in these worthy objectives need to have a grasp of the basic biology of the pig. An understanding of pig flow round the whole unit is important since this will have a major influence on the stresses and opportunities imposed upon the pig by the system itself. A shortfall in pig places generally presents itself as a compromise in managing the pig's environment. The space provided for the pig must meet its changing needs, taking account of the system of feed allocation and welfare requirements. Simple calculations must be undertaken so that all the physical interactions get the required response.

The uniqueness and harshness of the pig environment must be acknowledged and the fact that within it the physical demands upon control equipment necessitate that it must be robust, of good quality and be installed by professionals. Non-specialised control equipment widely used in general industrial situations is often short-lived when introduced to the challenging environment of the pig farm. Rather than be regarded as an expensive addition to a substantial but separate outlay of capital, environment control apparatus must be regarded as a worthwhile investment in a production plan that will yield a measurable payback. Staff must be trained to regard such installations as an essential part of their working tools to be used to help nurture the pigs in their care and so generate profit. The labour force must be trained to check themselves by monitoring the pig environment regularly and accept that excellence is more likely to be achieved if there is independent checking of the results of their actions. This book should not be regarded as a plea for fine-tuning but more of a reminder of the importance of setting-up the basics correctly and ensuring that they continue to be provided. Best practice is rarely achieved by chance.

Monitoring can take on many forms. Even when a pig building has the benefit of state-of-the-art control systems, the pig keeper must always assume overall ownership of the environment in which the pigs are housed. Opting out and allowing technology to take care of all key decision-making is not acceptable for those entrusted to work in modern, industrialised pig keeping systems.

Within the United Kingdom, the Code of Recommendations of Livestock – Pigs stresses the need to staff pig units with sufficient personnel possessing appropriate knowledge and professional competence (Defra, 2003). The document states that the stock keeper has the most significant influence on the welfare of the pigs. The Welfare of Farm Animals (England) (Amendment) Regulations 2003 (S.I. 2003 No. 299), Schedule, 6, Part II, paragraph 2, requires that: "All pigs shall be inspected by the owner or keeper of the pigs at least once a day to check that they are in a state of well being". The Code goes on to mention that stock keepers must be familiar with the normal behaviour of the pigs and it stresses that stock-keepers must have sufficient time to:

- Inspect the stock,
- Check equipment, and
- Take action to deal with any problem.

There is a chasm between merely meeting the welfare needs of pigs and maximising efficiency of production. Now the ability of the stock keeper to recognise abnormal pig behaviour and assume a more pro-active approach is being enhanced by the sensible use of modern technology. Quality assurance schemes demand that pig buildings should have maximum/minimum thermometers available to help stock keepers meet their objectives. Those routinely committed to taking daily temperature readings will, at least, have some understanding about the degree of temperature fluctuation and use this as a basis for decision -making with respect to environment amelioration. However, room temperature is only one element of pig environment. Technology has moved on and modern pig keepers must embrace this technology and use it to supplement their stock-keeping skills. This is a book for perfectionists, those with an enquiring mindset. The authors hope to motivate pig people who typically ask:

- Do I understand the biological needs of the pig?
- Does the environment I have provided meet those basic needs?
- How am I doing now?
- How does this compare with previous achievements?
- Can I do any better?
- How should I tackle the challenge of making changes that will bring about improvements?

"*Perfecting the Pig Environment*" draws on the experience of 'early adopters' who have made much use of technology as a means of making pigs feel more comfortable and boosting the profits of those who keep pigs. It helps define best practice and encourages its uptake for the benefit of pigs, pig keepers, processors, retailers and consumers. The book demonstrates what able stock people already know, that the most productive pigs are those attentively nurtured within a health and welfare conscious regime.

ENVIRONMENTAL MONITORING – THEORY, COMMON PRACTICE AND BEST PRACTICE

'Hit and miss' management

Controlled environment pig housing is often little more than an act of faith. Simply assuming that the optimum environment is being provided 24 hours a day cannot be described as best practice in a modern pig industry striving to improve efficiency. Often there is a great chasm between what is actually happening in a pig environment and what is meant or thought to be happening.

Continuous monitoring of environmental conditions to detect problems, and taking prompt remedial action, must be regarded as an integral part of the awesome responsibility facing pig keepers. This more precise approach to management has become routine practice among glass-house growers and more recently the poultry industry and has, in this respect, shown the pig industry the way forward. Just as modern pig diets are meticulously formulated and routinely analysed to ensure consistent quality, so must the environment in which pigs spend their life. Systematic monitoring of pig environment is a fundamental component of quality control. Attention to detail is vital.

Introducing technology to monitor the pig environment

As the pig industry has needed to become more efficient, various monitoring devices have been employed to help stockpersons make more objective commercial decisions, particularly when reacting to the behavioural changes of pigs in their care. Reference to a basic thermometer informed pig keepers about the actual air temperature around a fixed point at any given time. Whereas a maximum/minimum thermometer measured actual temperature and extremes of temperature around a fixed point, it did little to inform the pig keeper about short-term temperature fluctuation within the house and the actual duration of the changing temperature regimes. Hand-held digital thermometers, whilst having the advantage of portability, were dependent on stockperson presence usually within the actual pig pen and this could lead to 'one-off' spurious temperature readings. The use first of cumbersome clockwork thermographs followed by more sophisticated, compact, battery-operated devices, delivered a fuller picture of diurnal temperature fluctuations about a fixed point. Multi-point data loggers then became available and were useful devices providing more comprehensive whole house data when used for short spells to help pinpoint particularly troublesome problems. Whilst these devices improved the overall knowledge of temperature and other environmental fluctuations within a pig building, their use was still very much a compromise. The temporary installation of these devices was awkward and time-consuming and they were too expensive to use on a routine basis throughout a range of different pig buildings.

Modern successful businesses need to deliver continuous improvement in all facets of their business. This can only be implemented if reliable information is available to decision makers. Once collated, it can be appraised to identify any causal relationships which either help or hinder the production system. Pig farmers must embrace this approach to drive their business forward, a typical improvement strategy has several stages:

DEFINITION

This involves the identification of an aspect of the management of the pig environment that has significant shortcomings. Once identified, a multi-disciplinary team is formed to tackle the problem. Some of the team members would be farm-based whilst others would be more detached from the problem and would bring specialist expertise such as veterinary or financial knowledge.

MEASURING

Preliminary data are collated to give an insight into how the production system is currently working. This helps give an early indication of the extent and possible cause of the problem and might help outline the type of remedial action necessary.

ANALYSIS

The preliminary ideas are used to help determine the reasons for the problems encountered. The various theories are then tested to help identify the real source of the problem.

IMPROVEMENT

The root causes of the problem are eliminated by means of developing appropriate design strategies and then implementing these so that shortcomings are overcome.

CONTROLLING

In order to reap the long term benefit of the improvement and stop the defect from recurring, new 'permanent' control features are introduced.

'State of the art' real-time monitoring

Whilst heuristics, i.e. human observations, must remain a vital aspect of pig environment management, in the future, as technology increases, its relative importance is likely to diminish. Proven heuristic rules can be processed electronically and used within computer-controlled automated systems which are able to make continuous use of information. Basically, heuristics is concerned with learning by investigation. Using technology as a monitoring tool must be regarded as an opportunity to enhance traditional human 'investigations' rather than replace them. Modern, state of the art monitoring, is non-subjective and can be undertaken without human interference twenty four hours a day. However, it provides a useful opportunity for pig keepers, owners and advisers to visit a particular site electronically, as frequently as desired, without negative impact on the behaviour of the pigs or without compromising their health status.

Given this more precise approach, this information can be used either to confirm the suitability of the pig environment or automatically implement any necessary changes. Future strategies, therefore, will require go-ahead operators to drive their businesses forward by identifying and relying upon intelligent systems that will generate commercially meaningful information.

This will help generate a mindset of continuous improvement and a desire to achieve a maximum return on the business investment.

In the last two decades, the development of reliable and low cost microprocessors has meant that automatic electronic monitoring systems have become both affordable and practical for continuous real-time use on pig farms.

Electronic data loggers can measure and record temperature, humidity, water flow, feed use, electrical consumption. Anything that can be measured can be recorded - so as to give an insight into production as it really happens. But it's important to bear in mind that some things are far more readily measured than others. It is easy and cheap to measure temperature and water use, for example, but expensive and difficult to measure pig weight in pen.

Pig farms are large installations, and data are only useful if they are gathered together. Older systems required that each sensor or reading be wired individually to a data logger - like a telephone system, where each house or office must be wired individually to the telephone exchange. This meant a lot of wiring and high cost.

Nowadays, sensors are wired to data gathering modules that communicate over a "shared" network. The most common type of network is multi-drop RS485. This typically allows up to 1 km of total network length, and up to 30 or more network "nodes". A node is a device that communicates on the shared cable, resulting in far lower installed cost than older "central unit" systems.

RS485 is, in fact, merely an electrical standard - defining the voltage and electrical signals on a single pair. For units to actually communicate (transfer data from one to another) a communication *protocol* is needed.

In principle, equipment from different manufacturers could be connected on the same network so it would be possible to have a single network on a farm that all equipment shared. In practice, there are so many different communication protocols that this doesn't work out. Even when two manufacturers use the same protocol, they tend to implement it slightly differently, so it's unusual - outside certain industrial-type applications for different makes to share an RS485 network.

The future of on-farm data networks may well lie with wireless technology. Eliminating long distance wiring could reduce installed cost considerably, though there are a number of challenges to be overcome before this becomes a reality. Wireless (radio) is a line-of-sight medium. Short distance one-to-one data links, such as from a bell-push to a door-bell, are cheap and easy, but longer distance many-to-many data links are more complex, and technology suitable for the distances and complexity required by pig farms is only now being developed.

At present, the most cost effective method for data-gathering on pig farms is by a "multi-purpose" wired network. That is, using a network for control and alarm and monitoring. As well as sharing use of the data network, this shares use of the microprocessor units, and the sensors. Since environmental issues are often related to how control systems are used, it also makes sense to gather data - such as settings - from the controllers and/or alarm units. Dicam® is the best-known example of a mutli-purpose data network in pig production.

Download and remote connection

Data loggers show current data readings, and some even have a limited display of past readings or summaries such as averages or max-min readings. However, the amount - and form - of such information is very limited, and for most purposes it's essential to download the stored data for analysis and presentation. Since the data is as likely - or perhaps more likely - to be used, or of interest, off- farm as on-farm, remote data download is recommended and often essential.
There are three main ways to download the data remotely -

• landline modem

• cellular

• broadband

Landline modem is sufficiently established as to be regarded as "traditional". In effect, a landline modem is a "cable replacement". The modems act as a "virtual cable" between a remote PC and a data logger. This kind of remote call requires exclusive use of the telephone line, and that can be a problem nowadays when farms want to use the same line for voice, fax, computer and other equipment such as feed system modems.

Cellular modems can be used in place of landline modems. The cellular network provides "pseudo-exclusive" use of the airwaves by multiplexing the radio frequencies, avoiding the issue of shared lines, but call costs can be high, and cellular modem connections are not universally available.

Broadband, as used here, means fast, "always-on" internet-type access - or TCP/IP. Broadband is the future, or perhaps the present, of modern communications. Broadband may work by landline, WiFi, GPRS or satellite - or a combination of any or all of the above. Broadband works by "packetising" data and transmitting/receiving it very fast.

The crucial point about broadband is not that data transfer is very fast as such - the actual amount of data to be transferred each day from a logging system is not particularly high. Rather, it is the fact of being "always on". That means there's no barrier to how often data is transmitted. This has a number of implications, opens a number of opportunities, but it will be some time before the pig industry - and other industries - fully wake up to them. One is that multiple systems can share the same "gateway" through a router. Data logging, Internet access, feed systems, voice calls, even video surveillance can share the same portal. Another is that certain types of processing and data tasks can be carried out just as easily remotely over the Internet as they can on the farm.

The application of modern technology is all too often hampered by the ability of on-farm staff to exploit it, due to lack of time and the necessary skills. Fast, remote access makes it possible to "outsource" certain skills more easily; for example, Barn Report - the market leader in real-time pig monitoring - is an example of cost effective outsourcing. Data logging, data management and presentation are managed remotely by experts, using a high degree of automated processing and specialist techniques that would be difficult for most farm staff to master. Yet the cost is less than that of an unskilled worker writing down max-min temperature readings once a day. Using landline connections, data has to be updated each day - partly due to call costs and connection delays. Broadband removes this kind of limitation, reducing costs and improving functionality.

Not many pig producers have broadband connections on production sites at present, for a number of reasons. Though one takes it for granted in towns, and costs continue to fall rapidly, landline broadband rollout is slower in rural areas, and some places may never get it because of technical limitations. However, WiFi broadband is available in many rural areas, and satellite broadband is available almost everywhere. Costs of these may be higher than landline broadband, but are still a tiny fraction of most production sites' incidental costs, such as electricity.

This novel approach begs the question *"Is the operator being monitored rather than the environment?"* At the best it would be regarded as an ally of the enlightened, committed in the battle to get the pig environment right. At the worst, it would become an uninvited objective reminder to those whose heuristic skills were lacking despite it trying to prevent operators from doing the wrong thing or not doing anything at all to the pig environment. Over time, technical knowledge would be accumulated regarding the provision of the most suitable environment for the pig; this knowledge then would be refined and help pinpoint the optimum situation for consistently high pig performance.

Is the traditional pig industry ready to embrace such Information Technology? A sideways glance at the poultry industry should convince pig people that increasingly they will have to compete within a global industry. International production and trade will continue and those with an established track record within the pig industry will have to confront the reality of international sourcing and international retailing. Previously protected markets are likely to become more accessible in line with the World Trade Organisation objectives. Technology will become a key determinant of competitiveness and there will be more innovation at an accelerated speed. Countries which are slow to adopt technology will place themselves at a competitive disadvantage.

In any industry, progress results from innovation and its take-up is governed by the willingness of early adopters to take on and refine new technology. (Figure 1.1).

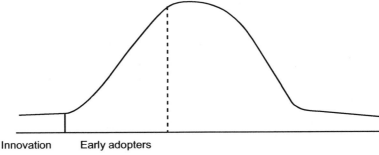

Innovation   Early adopters

Figure 1.1 The take-up of technology

Who will be the early adopters?

In particular, Information Technology knows no national boundaries. Although countries with a tradition of pig keeping have advantages of expertise, these industries are often burdened by an unwillingness to change and the existence of tired buildings and outdated plant and machinery which have become a barrier to progress. Traditional producer countries will have to undergo radical change if they are to compete within a global context.

Entrepreneurs in countries with emerging pig industries have little interest in outdated approaches to pig production. These global operators focus on 'state of the art' technology and install the very latest systems. This results in technological 'leap-frogging' and the trend will accelerate as suppliers increasingly focus on those who are most receptive to harnessing technology. Turnkey operators faced with a business plan and a clean sheet of paper have a refreshing mindset. Those setting up shop in places such as Brazil, Russia, Poland and the Asian Pacific region cannot afford to ignore the new opportunities that I.T. offers.

There is often a gaping chasm between those who are comfortable with 'computer-speak' and those who are most in need of boosting their businesses with new technology. Not only are the latter often unaware of new developments, their associated capabilities and an understanding of the potential to increase profits, there is also a training need relating to the exploitation of such opportunities on busy commercially focussed pig farms.

First pig farmers must get a better understanding of the optimum climatic environment for healthy pigs and profitable production; that was, and remains, the key objective of our previous publication *'Pig Environment Problems'*, Smith & Crabtree, 2005. Once a better understanding has been developed between the biological limitations of the pig and how the climatic environment impacts on them, the door to increasing profitability by using I.T. to identify key performance indicators may be opened. Better ways, therefore, have to be found of encouraging pig professionals to accept more ownership of the performance and lack of performance of the pigs in their care. Not only is this respectful of the needs of the pigs, but it enhances their welfare in accordance with the wishes of many consumers.

Figure 1.2 is a model representing how all those within the pork chain might better work together to ensure that Information Technology can be harnessed for the benefit of the whole of the pig industry.

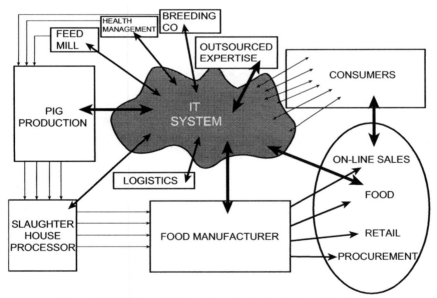

Figure 1.2 The future of information technologies in the pork food chain

Delivery will necessitate a degree of training input if only to make producers aware of the need and the potential of I.T. Just as profit-conscious pig farmers buy in expertise from those with specialist knowledge in pig health, in the future it seems likely that out-sourced expertise will be used to help keep abreast of new developments in technology and help ensure that those employing it achieve the very best commercial benefit throughout the changing life of pig buildings and the environment control systems within them.

Those prepared to out-source environmental monitoring would be freed from the burden and distractions of data collection. Recorded information would become available and accessible at all times; it could be used to motivate those responsible for running automated pig keeping systems and provide a focus for staff training sessions. When interpretation difficulties arose, telephone contact with an environment specialist would enable an early resolution of problems or misunderstandings. Operators would be provided with regular reports and so increase the likelihood of optimum performance from the installed system being achieved. It would be possible to identify and quantify 'normal' operational standards for a particular building and compare these to industry averages. Regular environmental monitoring would be used as a basis for fine-tuning control systems and reduce the rate of decline in efficiency as equipment deteriorates. Problems which build up as a result of water leakage could be minimised because these shortcomings would be identified at an early stage. Furthermore, water data could be used pro-actively as a basis for maximising pig health. Another advantage arising from ongoing I.T. monitoring would be the early identification of any disruption to feed supply. There would also be opportunities for reducing energy waste.

A venture into more sophisticated environmental monitoring can be likened to peeling an onion. There are far more layers than anticipated and the undertaking resembles a journey into the unknown, revealing well hidden but potentially vital information. The knowledge uncovered often contradicts and invalidates any preconceived ideas about the reasons for shortcomings in pig performance. It is a strategy more suited to those with enquiring minds rather than the headstrong. Sometimes shortcomings are identified which reflect misuse of a well designed building. On other occasions, the problems are attributable to climatic extremities beyond the building which arises because of the vagaries of the weather. Usually any resultant problems within the building are a reflection of poor management or hidden inadequacies in the design specification of the building.

The enlightened pig industry is on a steep learning curve and faces the challenge of harnessing IT and converting detailed and up-to-date knowledge of the pig environment into increased profits for the business. The following pages aim to help readers ascend the learning curve and confront the associated challenges. In most instances the information presented has resulted from case study work on commercial pig units where there is a professional focus on improved pig performance.

2

THE IMPACT OF STOCKING DENSITY – PIGS GENERATE HEAT AND INCREASINGLY NEED SPACE

Fundamental to the welfare requirements of pigs are the "Five Freedoms" which provide a logical basis for assessing those welfare requirements. The Code of Recommendations for the Welfare of Livestock: Pigs (DEFRA 2003) lists the Five Freedoms:

1. Freedom from hunger and thirst
   - *by ready access to fresh water and a diet to maintain full health and vigour.*

2. Freedom from discomfort
   - *by providing an appropriate environment including shelter and a comfortable resting area.*

3. Freedom from pain injury or disease
   - *by prevention or by rapid diagnosis and treatment.*

4. Freedom to express most normal behaviour
   - *by providing sufficient space, proper facilities and company of the animals' own kind.*

5. Freedom from fear and distress
   - *by ensuring conditions and treatment to avoid mental suffering.*

Provision of adequate space for growing pigs helps ensure that the Five Freedoms are met. If there are insufficient pigs in a pen, very likely they will be unable to generate sufficient heat to maintain the pigs above their lower critical temperature. The likelihood is that they would lie dirty and deplete their energy reserves simply in an attempt to keep warm. If there are too many pigs in the space provided, the surplus heat generated within the given pen area will have to be dissipated and this might well be beyond the capacity of the installed ventilation system. Vices would be likely to develop, feed and water intake would be erratic and there would be a wide variation of body weights within each pen. It is crucial, therefore, that when buildings are planned or production systems modified, that due attention is given to the issue of space allowance.

Knowledge of the changing floor area requirements of growing pigs helps reduce the likelihood of pigs running out of space and their welfare and productivity being compromised. The Code of Recommendations for the Welfare of Livestock: Pigs (DEFRA, 2003) refers to the provision of unobstructed floor area available to each weaner or growing pig and states a minimum allowance.

a.   0.15m² (1.6 ft ²) for each pig where the average weight of the pigs in the group is 10kg (22lb) or less.

b.   0.20 m² (2.5ft²) for each pig where the average weight of the pigs in the group is more than 10kg (22lb) but less than or equal to 20kg (44lb).

c.   0.30m² (3.2 ft²) for each pig where the average weight of the pigs in the group is more than 20kg (44lb) but less than or equal to 30kg (66lb).

d.   0.40m² (4.3 ft²) for each pig where the average weight of the pigs in the group is more than 30kg (66lb) but less than or equal to 50kg (110lb).

e.   0.55m² (5.9 ft²) for each pig where the average weight of the pigs in the group is more than 50kg (110lb) but less than or equal to 85kg (187lb).

f.   0.65m² (7ft²) for each pig where the average weight of the pigs in the group is more than 87kg (187lb) but less than or equal to 110 kg (242lb).

g.   100m² (10.8 ft²) for each pig where the average weight of the pigs in the group is more than 110kg (242lb).

The total floor area provided should be adequate for sleeping, feeding and exercising. The lying area itself must be sufficient to allow all pigs to lie down together on their sides without any incursion into the dunging area.

Prior to embarking on monitoring procedures dependent on utilising I.T., fundamental questions relating to the changing space requirements of housed pigs must be methodically addressed. Since pigs need increasing space as they grow, there has to be a practical compromise. It is, however, essential that when pigs first enter the pen and when they are about to leave the pen, inappropriate space provision must not compromise their comfort zone.

Back to basics

A case study from a commercial farm helps illustrate the point. A building originally designed to house pigs from 7kg (15 lb+) to 30kg (66lb) was re-assigned to house pigs from 15kg (33lb) to 40kg (88lb). Originally, by the time pigs left the building when averaging 30 kg (66lb), a nominal lying area of 0.3m² (3.2ft²) per pig was provided.   Additional to this minimum requirement, space was allocated for exercise and feeding *etc.* on the basis that 15% of the total floor area would be needed for these activities. Given a total pen floor area of 300m² (3229 ft ²) calculations suggested a maximum stocking density of 850 pigs at 30kg liveweight. In practice, typically 780 to 800 pigs were allocated to the space and the system worked well. Assuming the 15% space allowance for exercise *etc.* was constant; calculations indicated that room capacity at 40kg (88lb) would be around 726 pigs or 637 pigs to 50kg (110lb).

Figure 2.1 indicates the actual minimum, maximum and average stocking rate over a recorded period, data points for days when the building was empty have been omitted from the chart.

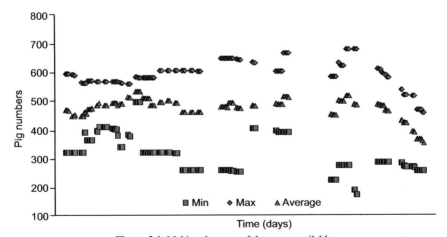

Figure 2.1 Making the most of the space available

Figure 2.1 helps explain why pig performance under the new stocking regime was disappointing. On average only 474 growing pigs were housed in the available space. Furthermore, during most of the time, well under 400 pigs were present. Although on occasions the stocking rate approached full capacity, for much of the time the building was stocked significantly below its capacity. A fundamental problem with this building was that regularly, when first stocked, low pig numbers failed to generate the temperature lift required. Pigs would feel cold in this building and the minimum ventilation rate would be above that recommended for the pigs housed.

Whereas the underlying theme throughout this publication is concerned with the potential that I.T. has for identifying shortcomings, the installation and deployment of sophisticated electronic measuring gadgetry is irrelevant if basic requirements have not been met. In this instance the primary need was to measure the effective space available within each room and decide on the most appropriate group size. A tape measure, weigh scales or even a good eye and some reference to published tables would have been a good starting point. Thereafter, bearing in mind the inevitable fluctuations in pig throughput that do arise in the real world, more effort was required in trying to ensure that the actual number of pigs housed was aligned more closely with the practical optimum. Until fundamental shortcomings such as space allocation, *i.e.* the physical environment have been addressed, there is little point monitoring climatic environment using either traditional or state of the art methods.

3

DATA INTERPRETATION – MAKING THE MOST OF ENVIRONMENTAL MONITORING

As the industry confronts the challenge of information technology, go-ahead pig people must not become victims of information overload. Interpretation of data-logger information generated during monitoring initiatives in pig buildings must not be allowed to overwhelm novice observers. This chapter focuses on simple example print-outs and aims to kick-start the thinking process of those committed to improving pig environments via systematic data logging. It is intended as a gateway to the interpretation of more complex case study work described in subsequent chapters.

The example chosen relates to recorded data from a fan ventilated finishing pig building accommodating 1000 pigs on slats. Pigs were dry fed from *ad-lib* hoppers automatically topped-up by augers. A single water meter recorded water use in the building and there were four feed augers, around 250 pigs were therefore fed from each auger. Feed delivery was measured simply by counting the number of seconds that the auger motor was running using a mains presence detector.

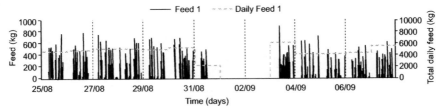

Figure 3.1 Total Feed Use and Individual Auger Runs

In Fig 3.1 individual spikes show each auger run. The auger was allowed to run as necessary to refill the hoppers, and typically ran about 6 to 10 times a day. The broken horizontal line represented the total running time each day. Since augers run as necessary to refill hoppers, and augers have a certain rate of delivery, the daily total run time was representative of how much feed was delivered. There was a big gap in the middle of the recording period when the auger did not run for several days. Since in-pen hoppers have some reserve capacity, it was not clear from this information whether or not pigs actually ran out of feed and whether, or to what extent the pigs may have been affected, and whether they were able to recover from this setback.

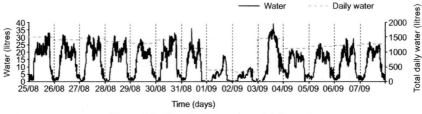

Figure 3.2 Water intake pattern and daily total

Fig 3.2 relates to water intakes and answers the foregoing questions in qualitative, if not quantitative terms. As with feed intake, there was a 'normal' pattern of water consumption - though in this instance, water flowed for much of the time, except at night. As before, the horizontal line shows the daily total. Water intake plummeted abruptly not long after the feed auger stopped running, and somewhat earlier than water intake dropped on previous days. This indicates that, in-pen feed hoppers did not hold much feed. During the next two days - when the auger did not run - water use was far lower. Without feed, these pigs still drank water, but obviously not very much.

On the day that the feed supply was restored, both feed and water intake were higher than before, however, during the following day both were lower than before, before climbing again.

The obvious point to make is that only those supplied with this information are in a position to do anything about it. Being a contract finishing building, the production supervisor might well have visited the farm and found the pigs without feed, in which case questions that should have been asked might well have included:

• How long had they been without feed?
• Why did it happen?
• Had production been affected?
• Had it happened before?
• Was it avoidable?

To which the answer might well have been that it was because the feed delivery lorry failed to turn up. However, this could have been regarded as a 'one off' incident; the pigs were not long without feed, and they would not have come to any harm, bearing in mind some pigs are restrict-fed.

A big advantage of electronic logging is the facility to widen the scope of any investigation. At the click of a button, in this instance, it is possible to answer some of the questions posed by investigating what actually happened over a four week period. This is shown in Figure 3.3. It indicates that there were two earlier interruptions to feed supply two weeks prior to the main incident. Although these earlier mishaps were not as disruptive as the main incident, again water intake was temporarily impaired. The reality was that within a matter of days, there had been an unacceptable disruption to feed supply on three occasions.

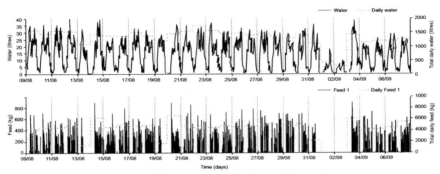

Figure 3.3 Water and feed intake over four weeks

No production data was available which would have enabled calculations to have been undertaken to help quantify the impact that these or any other incidents- may have had on growth, health or efficiency. The pig unit supervisor was aware that productivity on this farm was poor, and these graphs helped pinpoint some of the reasons. However, even the very best pig keepers are unable to solve problems before they have been identified.

4

TEMPERATURE MONITORING – A GOOD STARTING POINT FOR FINE-TUNING THE PIG ENVIRONMENT

Pigs will thrive provided they are housed within their 'zone of thermal neutrality'. However, the biology of the pig is such that although it might be comfortable when kept within a certain temperature regime, it might not necessarily be commercially productive (Smith & Crabtree, 2005). On many pig units, room temperature monitoring is confined to the automatic notification of equipment failure which can rapidly lead to the Upper Critical Temperature (UCT) being exceeded. In temperate regions, economics demand that modern pigs are housed just above their Lower Critical Temperature (LCT). If room temperature falls below this requirement, a disproportionate amount of feed will be used to keep the pig warm and body tissue may be broken down to help achieve this objective. If the temperature becomes too high, normally well before the UCT barrier has been breached, pig feed intake will be impaired and this will impact negatively on the efficiency of pig production.

In commercial situations, room temperature is set at a recommended target level which, amongst other things, is influenced by the quantity and quality of feed provided. However, it is also influenced by factors such as the incidence of draughts at pig level and the characteristics of the lying area, including the effectiveness of any bedding supplied. Whereas efficiently run pig systems owe much to the suitability of the average set temperature, pigs respond adversely to extremes of temperature and rapid temperature variation. Those entrusted to run modern pig units need to know how close actual room temperature is to that targeted and the extent of the variation. This is the very reason why on-going room temperature monitoring can help improve efficiency.

Temperature control in naturally ventilated buildings

In naturally ventilated pig buildings where there is only limited scope for controlling air movement, selecting and maintaining the optimum temperature assumes great importance. Whilst observing the automatic opening and closing of ventilation flaps on buildings fitted with Automatic Control of Natural Ventilation (ACNV) might be reassuring, it does not guarantee that the building is being run at the selected optimum temperature. Regular checking of the ventilation controller and ventilation flap actuators should be integrated into the management protocol of the building.

Particularly during late spring and early autumn, problems can arise when there is a wide variation between the extremes of day and night ambient temperature. When day time temperature is moderately warm, ventilation flaps will open. If they have not been set-up properly, such that the flaps are slow to react, when ambient temperature falls at night, very likely the pigs will feel cold. Particularly in finishing buildings, *i.e.* where much body heat is dissipated, during hot summer weather ventilation flaps necessarily remain open for long periods. In effect, under these circumstances, the inside temperature is being governed by the outside temperature and so the sensitivity of the controller is not particularly relevant.

At the onset of autumn and winter, however, the sensitivity of the controller settings becomes crucial. If the ventilation flaps were too slow to react to lower ambient temperatures, the comfort of the pigs would be compromised and very likely their respiratory health would be impaired.

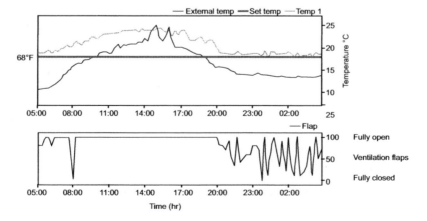

Figure 4.1 Daily temperature fluctuation in pig finishing building with ACNV

Figure 4.1 represents a situation where an ACNV system just happens to be working well but has actually been badly set up. The set temperature was 18°C (64.4°F) and during a 24 hour period the actual room temperature stayed reasonably close to the set temperature, but was obviously governed by the external temperature and wind speed.

The lower graph in Figure 4.1 depicts the degree of opening and closing of the ventilation flaps. It indicates that during the day when the temperature could be influenced by the prolonged opening of the ventilation flaps, temperature control was as good as practically possible, *i.e.* the flaps remained fully open and within the limits imposed by the high outside temperature, they did their job. However, as the outside temperature fell at night time, the ventilation flaps were continuously opening and closing and this led to unhelpful temperature fluctuation.

Figure 4.2 shows the same building in which the controller had been set up to be more closely aligned with the needs of the pigs.

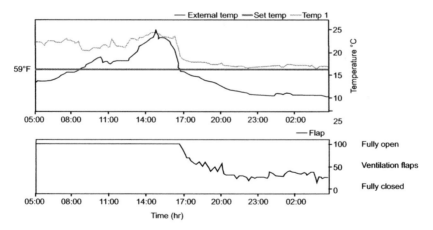

Figure 4.2 ACNV building with better control

In this instance, the set temperature was 15°C (59°F). During hot daytime conditions, as before, the ventilation flaps fully opened in an effort to get more air through the building. However, the fine top line depicting room temperature has fewer ripples at night time compared to the same time period in Figure 4.1. This arises because the degree and frequency of opening of the ventilation flaps was reduced and so the extremes of air flow were avoided during the cooler night time conditions. This significant improvement was attributable to the fact that the controller had been set to a wider *proportional band*. This facility within the controller determines how much movement it will trigger when the actual room temperature deviates from the set temperature.

In Figure 4.1, the proportional band had been set to 1°C. The significance of this setting was that for every 0.1°C deviation from the set temperature, it was making a 10% change in flap position, *i.e.* a significant amount of movement. In Figure 4.2 the proportional band had been set to 3°C. That means there was only a 3.3% change in flap setting for every 0.1°C temperature deviation from the target for the building.

Paradoxically, this favourable outcome has actually arisen because the controller has been made to be less sensitive, rather than more sensitive. If ACNV controllers are set-up to be highly sensitive, that is how they behave, *i.e.* they trigger an early reaction to deviations from the target temperature. In other words, they overreact in a futile attempt to generate a 'quick fix'. If, however, the flaps have been opened more than actually necessary, then they have to move back and the sluggish nature of linear actuators which open and close the ventilation flaps is such that they take a long time getting them to their destination. Whereas target temperatures are important, in many practical situations, stable temperatures are probably more important.

ACNV systems do not demand much energy input. However, if temperature bands are set wider, energy consumption would be reduced. Furthermore, the fact that the ventilation flaps open and close less, helps reduce wear and tear. Hence there are several good reasons for ensuring that ACNV systems are set up to perform over a wide proportional band. Avoidance of mechanical wear is a significant issue with curtain-sided buildings which often depend on winches and pulleys. These deteriorate with constant use, so in the interests of efficiency it is good practice to minimise their use and at the same time help generate a more stable temperature within a building.

Failure to achieve temperature lift – a case study

A monitoring exercise within a straw-bedded finishing building accommodating pigs from 40kg to slaughter pinpointed the impact of low stocking rates, poor wind resistance and the minimum ventilation rate set too high. Data relating to a five day period is shown in Figure 4.3

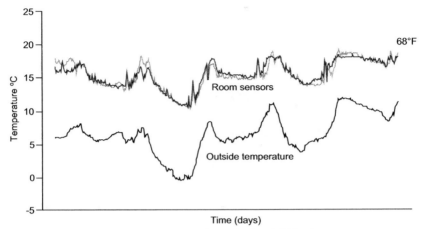

Figure 4.3 Air temperature fluctuation in a finishing house

It is apparent that temperature control within the pig building was poor and was greatly influenced by the outside temperature. Effective control was only achieved on day five. On that day the two sensors within the building then indicated much less temperature fluctuation than in previous days and room temperature kept close to 18°C (64.4°F). The record of outside temperature shown on the graph indicates that by day 5 the ambient temperature kept close to 12°C (53.6°F). In effect, better control was achieved inside the building as a result of day five being warmer outside the building. Room temperature tended to track the outside temperature in this badly managed building. However, the fall in temperature within the building was not as great as that recorded outdoors.

Figure 4.4 refers to a whole month of data relating outside temperature to the average inside temperature and also shows the temperature lift (T lift) above the outside. As the outside temperature falls, the inside temperature falls but the temperature lift increases. Mathematically this approximates to:

$$\text{T lift} = 12.3 - (0.47 \text{ x external temperature})$$

Consequently, when it is freezing point outside, the temperature lift is 12.3°C (54.1°F) but this lift diminishes when the outside and inside temperatures increase. Put another way, when it is cold outside, heat is necessarily produced within the building.

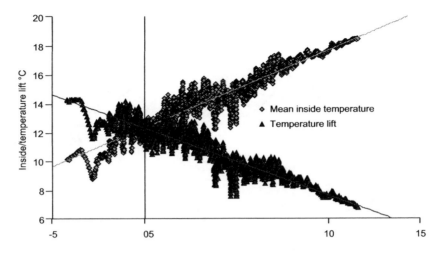

Figure 4.4 Changes in temperature and temperature lift

There are several possible sources for this heat:

- Thermal mass of the building.
- Solar gain.
- Less wind effect, *i.e.* heat *loss* is reduced.
- More heat is generated from the pigs themselves.

If the temperature within the building were lower, then there would be a bigger difference between the air temperature inside the building and the actual temperature of the building structure. This thermal gradient would result in the structure losing more heat. Since the blockwork building provided some insulation it tended to resist temperature falls and resisted temperature rises. Therefore, there was a thermal lag associated with the building.

Studies undertaken on empty buildings, *i.e.* those with little or no ventilation and heat removal, suggest that the extra heat output cannot be attributed to the building structure. Furthermore, meteorological records indicate that within the United Kingdom wind speeds tend to be lower at lower temperatures, hence higher wind speeds are a feature of milder UK winter weather. This could well explain some of the variability of the temperature trace but it does not seem to be a major factor. In the monitoring exercise reported in Figures 4.3 and 4.4, predictably the very lowest temperatures tend to be recorded at night. This diminishes the likelihood that the extra temperature lift arose because of solar gain. The probability is, therefore, that the extra temperature lift resulted from increased heat output from the pigs themselves, since they sensed the need for a warmer environment. Whilst this could be described as a useful biological adaptation, there is cause for concern. Heat is most certainly produced as a result of metabolism and activity. However, when extra heat has to be produced involuntarily there is a commercial conflict which could degenerate into a conflict with pig welfare. It is an energetically expensive process rather than the 'free' heat dissipated as a result of normal metabolism within the comfort zone. If the operator of a defective pig building such as that described is made aware of its shortcomings at an early stage, there is an opportunity to impose some cost-effective remedial action. If environment monitoring is not undertaken the likelihood is that mediocre performance would endure and not be questioned until either a serious health problem or economic loss become apparent.

Justifying capital expenditure on creep lamp temperature control

Regular temperature monitoring does not necessarily indicate shortcomings in an environment. It can, however, be used to confirm that an existing investment in environment control is giving the anticipated financial payback. Armed with this information, further similar investments can be made with increased confidence. A year long creep lamp monitoring exercise on a 2550 sow breeding unit indicated the justification of controlling their electricity uptake. Lamps rated at 125 watts (426.5 Btu/hr) were suspended over open creeps in 18 farrowing rooms each housing 24 crates.

The heating pattern shown in Figure 4.5 refers to one room monitored over a three month period. A feature of the graph is the cyclical nature of heater use over successive farrowing batches.

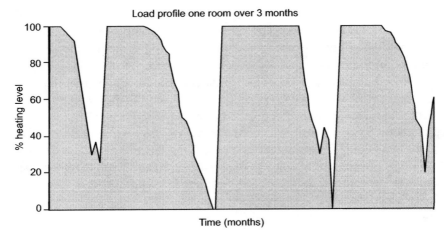

Figure 4.5 Creep lamp use in a farrowing room

Age of litter and ambient temperature have a major impact on creep heating demands. However, the data recorded in Figure 4.5 reflects the fact that the cyclical impact due to litter age was not a factor since the throughput pattern brought with it a wide range of litter ages within the room. In this instance, therefore, ambient temperature was the key influence on the demand for heat lamp use.

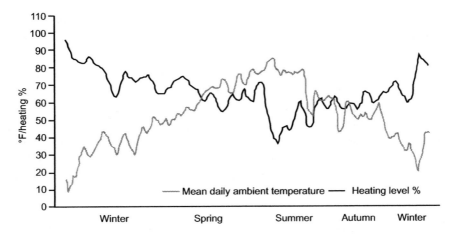

Figure 4.6 Ambient temperature, creep temperature and heater usage

Figure 4.6 indicates that more supplementary heat was used when the outside temperature was lowest. The mean ambient temperature averaged 11.7°C (53°F) over the year.

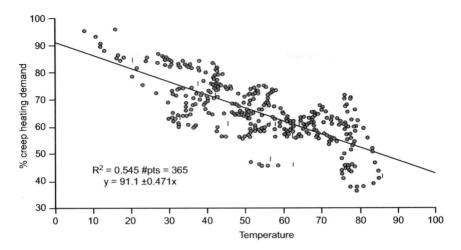

Figure 4.7 Correlation between creep heating demand and ambient temperature

Figure 4.7 shows the regression line which indicated an average reduction in creep heating of 0.47% per °F ambient daily temperature above -20°F on this U.S. based pig unit. Using average ambient temperature figures and the regression equation, calculations indicate that the theoretical average creep lamp use should have been 66.1%. The average use actually measured was 65.6%, *i.e.* reassuringly within 1% agreement.

On this large breeding unit, creep heating costs averaged 5.48 kWh (17.3 Btu/hr) per pig produced. Calculations indicate that if the creep lamps had not been controlled, heater use would have been 8.07kWh (25.4 Btu/hr) per pig and the average annual heating demand would have been 66.8% of the maximum available.

The creep lamp temperature controllers were therefore responsible for a saving of around a third. The savings potential would have been greater if the creeps had been covered. However, on large breeding units there is often a trade-off between ease of observation and energy costs. The key issue was that the pig farmer was able to quantify the benefit from capital invested in a specific aspect of environment control and justify further similar expenditure in the future.

The foregoing case studies highlight the impact that room temperature can have on pig productivity. They also demonstrate that average temperatures and historical maximum/minimum temperature readings are of limited value on efficient finely-tuned pig units. Continuous temperature monitoring provides an early indication of whether target temperature readings are being achieved and whether the degree of temperature fluctuation is compatible with good pig health and cost-effective production. On-going monitoring can also help determine whether or not control equipment has been set up properly and is appropriate for varying ambient conditions. It also provides a means of evaluating the cost-effectiveness of capital expenditure intended to ameliorate the environment and reduce costs. On-going monitoring is the management tool which confirms normality and provides an early warning of abnormality.

5

VENTILATION – THE ULTIMATE PRACTICAL COMPROMISE

The impact of changing ventilation rates

On commercial farms there is a tendency to alter ventilation rates based on human observations rather than scientific principles. Great reliance on 'the experienced pig keeper's nose' is still a feature of modern pig farming and often such reliance is overplayed. Whilst some human noses might be able to detect the presence of odours, most are not very good at actually measuring the concentration of the associated noxious gases. Few noses could differentiate between, *e.g.* 30ppm of ammonia and 10ppm in a way that would enable meaningful adjustments to be made to the ventilation controls.

Not only is the human olfactory system poorly equipped for measuring concentrations of noxious gases, people generally have little experience of comparing air quality on different farms. Furthermore, sensitivities differ and someone might regard any smell of ammonia as excessive whilst others would be prepared to tolerate levels in excess of 20ppm, *i.e.* above what many regard as the upper limit. If a subjective assessment suggested that ammonia concentration was 25ppm and this turned out to be right, what could be done to improve air quality to 20ppm ammonia or lower? This would involve a 20% reduction in ammonia concentration and would require a 20% increase in the ventilation rate. In other words, if a fan were set to give a minimum ventilation rate of 10% of the fan's maximum capacity, it would have to be increased to 12% to clear the 'excess' ammonia. In effect a 450mm (18 ins) diameter fan operating at a minimum ventilation rate of 500m³/hr (295ft³/min) would have to be adjusted so that the ventilation rate increased by 20%, i.e. it would need winding up so that it removed 600m³/hr (355ft³/min). The practical reality is that increasing the ventilation rate will not have an *immediate* impact on ammonia levels. If 500m³/hr (295ft³/min) brings about five air changes per hour, *i.e.* once every 12 minutes, it would take 5 x 12 minutes = 1 hour before ammonia levels reached the lower level of 20ppm. Most operators anticipate that the air quality would be restored in a much shorter interval of time. When this does not happen, the typical human reaction is to increase the ventilation to double this amount so that they are more quickly able to sense the impact of their intervention. Unlike the pigs, people do not remain in pig buildings and the chances are that this adjustment will soon result in over-ventilation when the operator is no longer present to make observations in the building.

Practical limitations

Is there an objective method of setting a more appropriate minimum ventilation rate? Generally, the minimum ventilation rate is required to provide an acceptable air quality, *i.e.* an environment in which there will be adequate removal of contaminants such as water vapour, dust and noxious gases. Throughout the world, the recommendation for maximum permissible levels of noxious gases varies considerably, *e.g.* ammonia upper limit recommendations vary between 10ppm and 50ppm depending on the country. Given this uncertainty, the basis for setting minimum ventilation is somewhat imprecise. Whereas there might be general agreement in the ventilation objective, what should design engineers and pig building operators actually do to achieve this is unclear.

As described earlier, depending on the human nose as the guide to setting minimum ventilation rate usually results in over ventilation, *i.e.* systems are made to operate far higher than theoretical models suggest. Young pigs with low body weights and low feed intakes necessarily minimise their heat loss. They live in an environment which not only needs the removal of noxious gases but also, on occasions, there is a requirement for heat input. On the other hand, in most situations, ventilation systems for growing and finishing pigs are designed with the objective of removing heat; the problem is, therefore, that the system has to cope with a wide range of ambient temperatures and a wide range of live-weights. In offices and factories it is much easier running a ventilation system at a constant level because body weight tends to be constant. Within the pig industry there is a trend towards fewer moves between buildings. This development, along with the tendency to slaughter lean, genetically improved pigs at higher live-weights exacerbates the problem of having to provide a wider range of ventilation rates. As pigs approach slaughter weight, particularly during hot weather, there is a need for a high ventilation rate. This need, however, is short-lived and for most of the growing and finishing cycle a much lower ventilation rate is appropriate.

A major challenge for ventilation engineers is to design systems with the appropriate 'competence'. This is defined as the ability to achieve a wide range of ventilation rates whilst maintaining good air distribution and even temperatures. In particular, there is a crucial requirement for the ventilation control to continue to be competent when the ventilation rate has to be set at a low percentage of the total capacity. Having said that, systems need not be over-specified. It is pointless designing systems that would work at as low as 1% of maximum capacity, when a 10% minimum ventilation rate would suffice.

Blending ventilation theory and practice

Design specifications providing a minimum ventilation rate which is 10% of the maximum capacity are commonplace. Fans set at lower speeds develop such low pressure that, despite the presence of protective cowls and baffles, they are easily overridden by wind pressure and so their effective throughput is both uncertain and inappropriate. Typically fan controllers allow ventilation rates between 100% and 10% of maximum running speed. It is not surprising, therefore, that the operators of pig buildings assume that the 10% setting provides the *correct* minimum ventilation rate. It might be right and it might not be right. In many situations the facility to vary ventilation rates between 100% and 10%, *i.e.* a 10 : 1 ratio would be adequate. The 10% setting sometimes, however, would not be sufficiently low to match the comfort zone of newly weaned pigs, particularly in situations where the ambient temperature was particularly low and/or weaning weights and numbers were below expectations. Such systems depend on supplementary heat input and so any degree of over-ventilation would be expensive. It is possible to achieve lower and more appropriate ventilation rates by:

- Using several fans, with two low output fans of equal size.

- Operating one of the low capacity fans at the 10% rate would allow the minimum ventilation rate to operate at only 5% of the minimum capacity.

- Using a combination of speed control and time-switching, *i.e.* an interval timer.

- Running a low capacity fan, *e.g.* for every five minutes in ten; setting such a fan to run at 10% minimum ventilation rate would actually achieve 5%.

- 'Throttling' a fan by means of automatic or manual baffles is another alternative.

As pigs grow, they eat more and produce more heat and so the minimum ventilation requirement increases. In effect they burn more fuel and a consequence of this metabolism is that they need to lose more water vapour and carbon dioxide which are the by-products of respiration. The need for this increased rate of ventilation is therefore governed by the extra quantities of water vapour and carbon dioxide produced. However, other factors might be more crucial, *e.g.* the level of gases in pig slurry, in other words what is below the slats could be more important than the body weight of pigs above them. Hence, the principle of increasing minimum ventilation rate with age, although practically convenient, may not be the correct course of action.

Increasing the ventilation rate also increases the degree of heat loss, besides clearing the air space of noxious gases. Put another way, it dilutes the concentration of the gases and dilutes the concentration of the heat energy within the building.

In practical terms, if the ventilation rate were doubled in an attempt to halve the concentration of contaminants, the temperature lift would be halved. Increasing a fan speed from 20% to 40% would reduce temperature lift from, *e.g.* 16°C (60.8°F) to only 8°C (46.4°F), so if the temperature were only 5°C (41°F) outside, it would just reach 13°C (55.4°F) inside. Hence, ventilation is a practical compromise which has to take account of many factors. These include outside temperature, wind effects, concentration of aerial contaminants within the building, pig bodyweight, heat production and the degree of insulation of the building.

Reasons why pig buildings are regularly over-ventilated

Pig building operators tend to set minimum ventilation rates too high. In nursery pens, since pigs of low bodyweight are particularly sensitive to low temperatures, the minimum ventilation setting is crucial because in these rooms it dominates air throughput for much of the time. There is usually much dependence on supplementary heat and so it would be uneconomic to operate with numerous regular air changes. Once pig body weight has increased and an *ad-lib* feeding is underway, air throughput has to be markedly increased. This transition from weaner to grower arises over a short period of time and in many instances operators lack training and fail to grasp the very different aerial requirements as the pigs eat and grow.

Maintenance of fan controllers is a neglected area on many pig farms and many 'first generation' controllers used in old buildings, although robust, were notoriously unreliable. Those responsible for pig production in these buildings distrusted automation of the ventilation control and tended to override them manually. The same mindset persists on modern pig units where there has been a failure to accept and benefit from the improved sensitivity of state of the art controllers. Human nature is such that in many instances blindly 'fiddling' with fan speed controllers has been regarded as the easy option rather than undertaking regular monitoring and using this as the basis for making changes to the ventilation settings.

Ad-lib fed finishing pigs have a wide comfort zone and in terms of pig welfare, their temperature is not crucial compared to younger pigs. Maybe this mindset dominates the thinking of those caring for more sensitive younger weaners. Another factor is that as finishing buildings age, the overall quality of the environment deteriorates. Respiratory diseases often then become a problem and air throughputs are increased in an attempt to minimise aerial contamination around the pigs. Again this is a 'hit and miss' management strategy and is no substitute for providing the optimum environment and monitoring to ensure all is as expected.

The design and operation of modern pig buildings often overlook 'the people factor'. Those who enjoy caring for pigs *per se* must not feel excluded from their management; automation must not devalue the important contribution made by people. When there are dials on environment control boxes, human nature, or maybe a genuine desire to get involved in improving the environment, results in people changing dial settings. On what basis do they make these crucial changes? In most instances there are two dials, one that alters the ventilation rate and another that alters the target temperature for the house. Adjusting the temperature setting eventually regulates the ventilation system but usually the response is not immediate. On the other hand, if the ventilation setting is adjusted, particularly if the minimum ventilation rate is increased, the stockperson observes an instant response. Fans speed up or ventilation flaps open and the perception of helpful intervention increases. The reality is that once the heat balance goes below that brought about by the revised minimum ventilation rate setting, temperature falls. Room temperature plummets below the target setting and will be further lowered by any subsequent drop in outside temperature. Temperature tends to be lower in the hours before dawn. The reality is that the foregoing scenario is likely to have its maximum impact when stockpersons are not around to observe the impact of their well-meant intervention. By the time people arrive for work, temperature is usually rising and could well be back to the target level. In the absence of systematic monitoring, there is no knowledge and no record of the environmental challenge suffered in the small hours; it could well have been the hidden trigger that started a costly health problem.

Case studies featuring over-ventilation

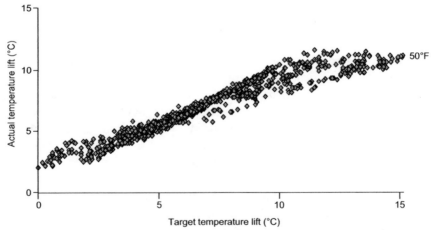

Figure 5.1 The relationship between temperature lift and ventilation rate

The graph shown as Figure 5.1 indicates a pig finishing situation, where on occasions, room temperature dips below the target level. This happens when it is particularly cold outside and the ventilation system is operating at its minimum capacity. On these occasions the inside temperature is only 10°C (50°F) above that recorded outdoors.

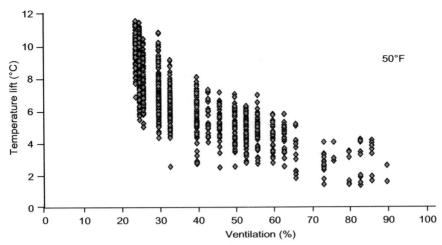

Figure 5.2 Over ventilated pig finishing house

Figure 5.2 depicts the relationship between temperature lift and ventilation rate. When the temperature lift is lowest, the ventilation rate is highest, *i.e.* the ventilation system is keeping the building cooler. However, in this instance, the minimum ventilation rate has been set at 25%. This is the reason why the temperature lift never increased once the minimum ventilation operated. If the minimum ventilation had been reduced, *e.g.* to 10%, then the temperature lift would have been greater, *i.e.* the minimum ventilation rate setting limited the capacity for temperature lift.

Figure 5.3 relates to data recorded over a two week period in a pig finishing house. The upper graph shows the room temperature and ambient temperature. The top two wavy lines depict room temperature readings. The straight solid line shows the target room temperature reading, whereas the fluctuating black line below it represents the outside temperature.

The lower graph is concerned with ventilation. The solid horizontal line shows the minimum ventilation setting and the wavy line shows the actual ventilation rate expressed as a percentage of the maximum. It can be seen that most of the time the top graph shows that room temperature remains close to the target. However, some of the time it rises by a few degrees. This happens when the ventilation system is operating near its maximum capacity. The maximum temperature reached in the house is governed by the ventilation capacity and the temperature lift of the system.

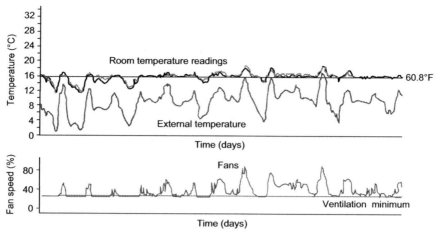

Figure 5.3 Temperature fluctuations and ventilation in a finishing house

In simple terms, the target temperature lift is the difference between the set temperature and the external temperature. Figure 5.1 shows the relationship between the *actual* temperature lift achieved and the temperature lift. When the target temperature inside needs to be 7°C (45°F) above that outside, *i.e.* towards the middle of the diagonal line on the graph, the relationship is linear. However, when the target temperature inside needs to be the same as that outside, the graph slope changes in that at 3°C (37°F) it becomes flatter. This temperature lift is the smallest possible and it cannot go any less because the ventilation system is working at maximum capacity. Towards the top end of the line on the graph it again flattens at about 10.5°C (50.9°F). This is because the system is not capable of creating a temperature differential of more than 10.5°C (50.9°F) between the outside and inside. In other words, when room temperature is between 3 and 10.5°C (37 and 50.9°F), the system is in control. When the required temperature lift is beyond this lower and upper limit, it is no longer in control, *i.e.* the system is severely limited. In other words, under these 'extreme' circumstances, outside temperature is the dominating factor. The inside temperature is only *modified* by the system rather than *controlled* by it.

The situation described arises because of the minimum ventilation control setting. Figure 5.2 indicates that the minimum ventilation rate was set at 23%. *i.e.* much higher than its potential minimum. Typically this situation arises when the operator of the building is concerned that ammonia levels would become excessive at lower ventilation levels. The real problem is not the ventilation system but more likely the design and management of the slurry disposal system.

Assuming that the ventilation capacity of the building is, *e.g.* 60 air changes per hour, if there are only 23% of these air changes, *i.e.* approximately 15 per hour, the result is excessive build up of ammonia, *i.e.* when air changes only once every 4 minutes (60 minutess ÷ 15). The reality is that in situations such as this, the building operator has made a fundamental decision, *i.e.* the setting of the minimum ventilation rate by depending solely on a poorly equipped human olfactory system. If science had been applied and actual ammonia levels had been measured at a range of low ventilation rates then a more appropriate setting for the minimum ventilation rate could have been established. In other words, the need for a lower minimum ventilation rate would have been scientifically established and there would have been an opportunity to exert more control over the environment of the building. By depending on the operator's nose which could well be super-sensitive to ammonia, the operator has subjected the pigs to episodes of insufficient temperature lift when outside temperatures are cold.

Figure 5.4 represents temperature variation in a second-stage weaner building.

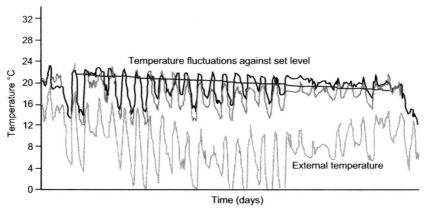

Figure 5.4 Temperature fluctuations in a second-stage weaner house

By the time the pigs are ready to leave the building they are less susceptible to temperature fluctuation and Figure 5.4 indicates reduced temperature variation with in it. There is a reasonable degree of control in that inside temperature is about 2°C (35.6°F) higher than that outside. However, when the room was first stocked and low outside temperatures arose, the temperature within the room was not adequate for sensitive newly moved weaners. On one occasion the minimum room temperature was as low as 11.8°C (53.2°F) *i.e.* most inappropriate for weaners. As it happened, the average temperature over the batch was 18.8°C (65.8°F) throughout a period when the selected set temperature was 20.1°C (68.2°F). Whereas the average temperature could be described as acceptable, on occasions the pigs in this environment would feel chilled to such an extent that health problems might arise.

The inevitable practical compromise

Given the shortcomings of the human olfactory system and the understandable tendency for pig carers to want to intervene, what is the best ventilation strategy in practice? In the real world there will be occasions when there has to be a trade-off between the need to run pig houses at the optimum temperature and the need to use ventilation to improve air quality by diluting aerial contaminants. Practical decisions have to be made. Does the person responsible for the welfare and productivity of the pigs:

- Maintain the target temperature regardless of air quality?
- Dilute aerial contaminants to an 'acceptable' level?
- Provide a compromise environment in which neither criteria are ideal?

Despite the plethora of research results and the degree of sophistication of the modern pig industry, nobody has the correct answer to this dilemma. The example shown in Figure 5.4 involved letting room temperature fall by more than 4°C (39.2°F) below what already was a low temperature target, or alternatively allowing a build-up of ammonia for a few hours. Since high levels of noxious gases are known to impair respiratory health, maintaining an aerial environment free from contaminants is recognised as good practice. However, as yet no research has measured the existence or extent of temporary exposure to marginally higher levels of noxious gases. Furthermore, experienced pig keepers observe that relatively small fluctuations in air temperature have a marked impact on pig behaviour. If this arises over a short period of time it need not seriously impair the thermal balance of housed pigs. There is, however, a degree of pressure on worthy pig keepers who observe pigs huddling or maximising their surface area to make changes to the environment in order to bring about more normal lying behaviour. Great importance is attributed to setting the minimum ventilation rate and never allowing it to drop below a certain value (10% in most instances). However, this has more to do with the avoidance of high wind speeds overriding fan motors rather than the proven needs of the pig.

Theory and practical experience suggest that in reasonably insulated pig buildings stocked at normal rates, the temperature lift resulting from body heat loss is sufficient to activate the ventilation system such that a reasonable air quality would prevail. However, when ambient temperatures are particularly low and pig weight or pig numbers are also low, there is justifiable concern that total dependence on conventional environment control settings could be short-changing the pigs.

Getting the best out of fans

Over the years, fans tend to deteriorate often from the inside out. Leaving fans not running for long periods in dirty and sometimes wet conditions does them no good. Wet fans are slow to warm-up and so struggle to dry out. In practice, fans in the same building often are subjected to widely different amounts of use. This is particularly so when first and second stage control is imposed. The outcome is that since they are used much more, first-stage fans need replacing long before second-stage fans. When first-stage fans wear out, it is common practice to replace them with existing second-stage fans or install new replacements. Over the years this can result in a building having a diverse mix of fans of different makes and ages. As a consequence there is every likelihood of fan failure arising at different times, often associated with unscheduled production setbacks and disproportionately expensive call-out charges for fan replacement or repair. A system which from the outset rotated fan use so that a more even wear pattern resulted would be more efficient. It would lessen the need for emergency call-out visits and increase the likelihood of implementing a more cost-effective strategy involving the replacement of fans of the same age and use pattern.

A facility known as 'Fan Switch' enables extraction systems incorporating two or more stages of identical fans to be rotated on a daily basis so that more even use patterns are imposed. The strategy involves the initial use of Fan 1 as the first-stage of ventilation (primary) and Fan 2 as the second-stage of ventilation (secondary). However, the system is set up such that on alternate days Fan 2 is used as the primary fan and Fan 1 is used as the secondary fan.

A FAN SWITCH CASE STUDY

The case study involved a pig farm with 19 nursery rooms housing pigs from weaning to 30kg. Each room had two identical extractor fans with 450 mm (18 inches) diameter. They were fitted with back-draught shutters, air entered via passive inlets and the study lasted for ten months. Rooms 1-15 used Fan Switch and Rooms 16-19 did not. Those without Fan Switch were set up so that Fan 1 was always used as the primary stage and Fan 2 as the secondary stage. Results for the 15 rooms with Fan Switch are shown in Table 5.1.

Table 5.1   Nursery rooms with Fan Switch Facility

Room number	Time weighted throughput of fans (%)		Average
	Fan 1	Fan 2	
1	27.9	28.2	28.1
2	31.0	31.7	31.4
3	33.1	33.2	33.2
4	28.7	29.1	28.9
5	31.6	32.6	32.1
6	31.1	30.9	31.0
7	31.6	32.2	31.9
8	33.0	33.5	33.3
9	29.6	29.7	29.7
10	29.2	29.3	29.3
11	26.9	26.9	26.9
12	26.3	25.8	26.1
13	32.1	29.1	30.6
14	28.7	30.7	29.7
15	27.7	26.6	27.2
Average of rooms 1-15	29.9	30.0	29.9

The data shows the average throughput of each fan as a time weighted average. This results, *e.g.* in a fan that revolved half the time at 20% speed and the other half at 40% speed and would show an average of 30% maximum capacity. The fans could either be switched off (0%) or have fully variable speed between 10 and 100%. In total, over a ten month period, 30,000 readings were taken for each fan. The speed as set by the controller was recorded every fifteen minutes. Minor differences in Table 5.1 arose because of small differences in the number of batches of pigs put through each room. The table clearly indicates, however, that with Fan Switch very even use was recorded on the two-stage system.

Results from Rooms 16-19 which did not have the Fan Switch facility are shown in Table 5.2.

Table 5.2 Nursery rooms without Fan Switch facility

Room number	Time weighted throughput of fans (%)		Average
	Fan 1	*Fan 2*	
16	47.9	7.7	27.8
17	53.3	10.2	31.8
18	53.0	10.9	32.0
19	49.8	7.1	28.5
Average of rooms 16-19	51.0	9.0	30.0

The table indicates that the first-stage fans were used five to six times more than the second-stage fans. Although the effective ventilation would be the same whether Fan Switch was in use or not, the delivery method was different. In rooms without Fan Switch, readings taken between September and February also indicated long periods without the second-stage being activated. In these rooms, wear on the fan bearings of the first-stage fans would be disproportionately high and they would be more likely to wear out years before the second-stage fans. Fan Switch provides an opportunity to manage events rather than crises.

6

FEED AND WATER – ALWAYS NEEDED BUT RARELY MEASURED

Modern pig farming involves the efficient conversion of feed and water into lean meat. Together they represent crucial inputs on what has essentially become a protein production line. The cost-effective production of lean meat is very much dependent on the ability to utilise feed and water to exploit modern genetics. Despite feed costs representing over 70% of variable costs and lean meat comprising over 70% water, many pig farmers have very little control over these inputs. Within any pig production system, the potential to control feed and water input increases markedly if their uptake is routinely monitored. It is a principle already well embedded in poultry production protocols and offers great opportunities to pig farmers who are ready to embrace this challenge.

The need is likely to increase as more cereal farmers choose to grow crops for the energy market and pig farmers find themselves competing on a rapidly changing world stage. Furthermore, water is becoming generally regarded as a scarce and more expensive resource. Hence, there are sound commercial reasons for establishing how much of this scarce resource is being taken up overall within the production system and how much of it actually reaches the intended target. Water monitoring, besides being helpful to farmers and pig unit managers, is also a useful diagnostic tool for consultants and veterinarians. Anecdotal evidence and clinical research indicates that the existence of some endemic diseases may be detected during the incubation periods by a reduction in water intake which can arise up to a week before signs of clinical outbreak of disease. When pigs are provided with natural lighting, typically their 'body clock' runs from about 6 a.m. to 6 a.m. This impacts on their behaviour and influences water intake patterns. Hence, when monitoring water intake in pigs, it is important to take measurements over a precise period which takes account of the body clock effects. One-off manual readings of water intake also fail to take account of variable and varying leaks within the plumbing system. Such readings are not sufficiently reliable to act, *e.g.* as a basis for the accurate administration of water-soluble drug treatment.

Using a data logger to record water intake from several reference points every 15 minutes, *i.e.* 96 readings per day, provides much more reliable information and allows both *total water intake* and *water intake patterns* to be accurately recorded. The pig industry is under much pressure to reduce medication levels and accurate monitoring of water intake helps achieve this objective. It also reduces the risk of pigs rejecting excessive levels of medication because of taint problems.

A case study indicating water shortage

This incident relates to a large finishing enterprise comprising 9,600 pigs in 24 rooms, each accommodating 400 pigs. Throughout the monitoring period, older pigs occupied Rooms 1 – 12 and younger pigs occupied Rooms 13 to 24. Figure 6.1 shows the trace of water intake for the older and younger pigs and is expressed in one minute intervals.

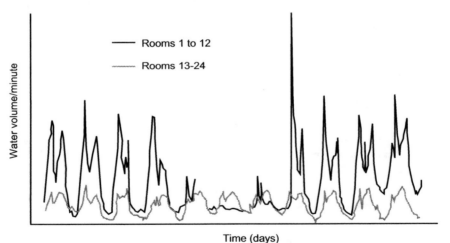

Time (days)

Figure 6.1 Water intake in finishing rooms

A discrepancy between intake patterns in the two finishing stages is most apparent. This arose because the water supply to Rooms 1 – 12 was disrupted; apparently a filter or pipe had become partially blocked with sand. Although some water remained available, the pressure and flow rate was lower than normal. Figure 6.1 shows the total consumption per minute for Rooms 1 – 12 and for Rooms 13 – 24, the consumption in each room has been added together.

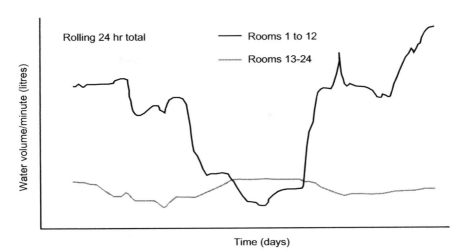

Figure 6.2 Average water intake per day in finishing rooms

Figure 6.2 shows the total consumption recorded per day. In Rooms 13 – 24, water intake remained steady whereas in rooms 1 – 12 it was somewhat variable, so much that the daily water intake in these rooms was less than half of that in the other rooms. The peaks recorded indicated an intermittent but recurrent problem, *i.e.* it was likely that blockages arose and then were temporarily cleared and this cycle kept repeating itself.

Eating and drinking tend to go together in pigs. Figure 6.3 relates to the duration of feed auger operation throughout the monitoring period.

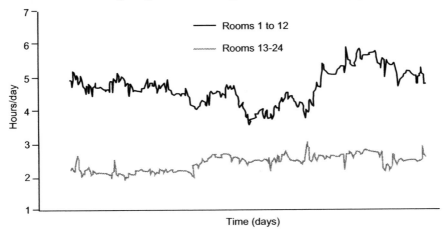

Figure 6.3 Daily hours of feed auger operations

On this unit, feed delivery via the augers was triggered by limit switches set to allow the auger to run a certain number of times each day. In Rooms 1–12, *i.e.* the rooms with the water supply problem, the auger running times were somewhat erratic. The peaks on the feed graph where nowhere near as pronounced as those on the water graph. This arises because individual augers run only a few times per day and do not necessarily coincide with actual eating times. This is the reason why the trace is not so obvious as with water which is intended to run all the time at the same rate.

Whereas in this instance feed use was not quite so depressed as it might have been, given the water supply disruption, it was still considerable and would impact significantly on feed conversion. If the feed intake was 1.5 times maintenance (1.5M), since 1.0M is used for maintenance, it would need two thirds of this intake just to maintain itself. In other words, a third reduction in feed intake would not allow any growth whatsoever.

It seems reasonable to assume that if water supply is disrupted, finishing pigs would choose to make good any deficit by spending longer taking in water. Figure 6.4 conflicts with this train of thought.

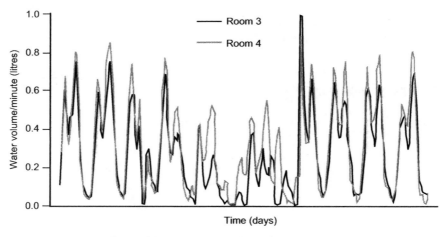

Figure 6.4 Water intake in adjacent finishing rooms

The figure indicates that the water intake pattern and total consumption in Rooms 3 and 4 which housed roughly the same number and age of pigs followed similar lines. The two lines on the graph are very much in phase in that the pigs drink at the same time. Room 3 seemed to be more affected by the water disruption problem than Room 4. However, overall the pattern and duration of water intake in the separate rooms was remarkably similar. Put another way, the pigs in the room suffering the most restricted water flow do just the same as those in a less troubled room. Either consciously or maybe subconsciously, they elect to drink water when it is available and invest little extra time looking for it when it is unavailable.

This incident arose on a commercial farm where it had proved necessary to remove some pigs from the rooms and this explains some of the shortfall in water uptake. However, this practical reality would not explain the prominent uptake surge recorded on 8 September when supply was restored to normal.

It is of some concern that during the early stages of the incident, those subjected to the disrupted supply chose only to drink as they might have done had water been in abundance. Water was still available, albeit at a reduced flow rate, but certainly during the first day of disruption finishers chose to leave it in the system rather than spend longer drinking. It seems likely that after about a day, pigs were more inclined to drink what they could, when it was available. A water intake pattern of peaks and troughs still persists but once the supply problem is rectified, the drinking habits of pigs in Rooms 3 and 4 become more synchronised.

This case study helped give the operators a better understanding of the drinking habits of pigs and the impact that a disruption of water supply might have on feed conversion. Pigs like to suckle together and they also like to eat and drink together. However, once their immediate nutritional needs are met, they only are prepared to spend a limited amount of time eating and drinking. The early indication of a disruption to water supply provides an early opportunity to make amends and help optimise feed intake and feed conversion efficiency.

A case study indicating a pig health problem

Figure 6.5 represents a situation where 2,000 contemporary pigs were weaned and moved to one of two wean to finish buildings. The pigs were genetically similar and had been raised in identical farrowing houses with the same management input. Figure 6.5 depicts differences in water intake patterns and total water intake in House 1 and House 2. After three days, in both instances, water intake was reduced, but this was most marked in House 1. Historical analysis of records on this farm indicated that the different intake patterns were very much associated with a change of diet. As is happened, there was a health problem in House 1 pigs and when the diet specification changed, these pigs reacted adversely to the change; this was reflected in reduced water intake. Following this health problem, pigs in House 1 continued to have lower water intakes than those in House 2. It was only after pigs had been removed from House 2 as they achieved slaughter weight that more water was being consumed in House 1 than House 2. Subsequent investigation indicated that feed intake had been impaired in House 1 which accommodated the pigs which had suffered a health check. If the graphs had been studied more closely, very likely the disease problem in House 1 pigs would have been spotted and early remedial action would have been taken. The situation described highlights the need to assess data-log charts and take appropriate action.

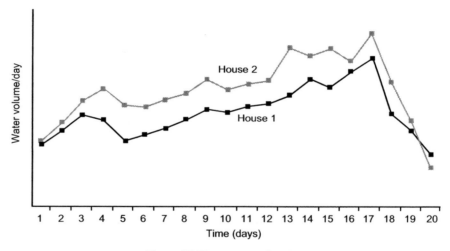

Figure 6.5 Water consumption chart

The importance of feed availability

Growing pigs use feed primarily for maintenance and any surplus is potentially available for growth. The maintenance requirement can be likened to a charge for overheads. It is simply the amount of feed energy the pig uses to replace spent energy and maintain its body tissues. If pigs only consumed their maintenance ration they would not grow and as pigs get bigger the overhead cost of maintenance increases. Commercial pig farmers cannot hope to make profits unless pigs achieve growth over and above the maintenance requirement. When pigs are young and have much potential for growth they are keen to consume much more than their maintenance requirement. As they get bigger they eat more food for maintenance but since their biological need for growth has diminished, it becomes increasingly difficult to get feed for growth into the pigs. Young pigs actually consume 5-6% of their body weight each day. As they get older and bigger, the daily feed intake reduces to 2-3% of their body weight and much of this food is partitioned into maintenance rather than growth. A simplified version of the concept is illustrated in Figure 6.6.

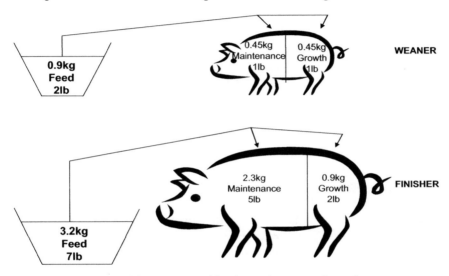

Figure 6.6 The partition of feed into maintenance and growth

The commercial reality is that if a pig is not fed for a day and extra feed is eventually made available, the maintenance deficit has to be replenished before any further growth can take place. Since this deficit in the maintenance requirement increases as the pigs get larger, the commercial consequences of missing out on feed intake become increasingly punitive.

The concept of pigs eating and drinking more after an episode of feed or water unavailability, *i.e.* catching-up for the earlier loss, is not valid. Pigs become accustomed to eating and drinking little and often. After being starved, they tend to gorge themselves to satiate their hunger. However, they cannot cope with sudden large quantities of food and digestive upsets result. This 'sickens' them and they react by eating less food until the gut well-being is restored.

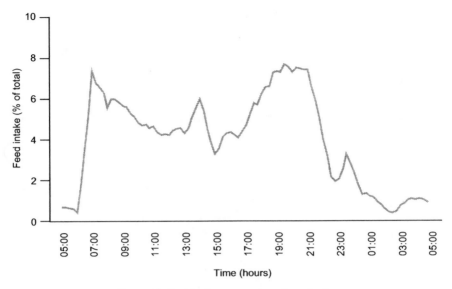

Figure 6.7 Feed intake patterns throughout the day

Figure 6.7 depicts a typical feed intake pattern throughout the day under high temperature conditions. The graph helps explain why feed deprivation at certain times of day can be more serious than at other times. It indicates that when the pigs wake up in the morning, there is a surge in feed intake. As the day progresses and the outside air temperature increases, feed intake is temporarily impaired. Later in the day when the cooler evening arrives, pigs become motivated to increase their feed intake. After sunset, feed intake diminishes again when pigs undertake a period of reduced activity. During the morning and afternoon periods of high feed intake, during each hour, 6-8 % of total daily feed intake is consumed. Feed delivery failures are never convenient but their impact is greatest when they coincide with periods normally associated with high intake. The right hand side of the graph indicates low feed intake during the hours of darkness. During the long interval between midnight and 6am only about 5% of the total daily intake is consumed. Hence, a feed delivery failure during that time interval would be less serious than at other times. In the example shown between 6pm and midnight, around 30% of the daily feed consumption was recorded. The peak intake between 7pm and sunset around 9pm actually represented around 15% of the daily intake. This probably arises because in their natural state, pigs choose to sleep after sundown. In order to see them through the period of night time inactivity, they choose to fill their guts with feed before settling down for the night. Sometimes, despite feed augers failing, intake of pig feed might not be impaired. This situation arises when there is an abundance of in-pen storage within sizeable feed hoppers. Sometimes feed intake monitoring may be 'confused' by counting time when an auger, although running, was not actually delivering feed. This situation can arise when feed bridges in the bulk bin. Occurrences such as this can be identified by comparing the daily total feed and water intake with days immediately before and after when the bridging problem was suspected.

Feed delivery failure incident

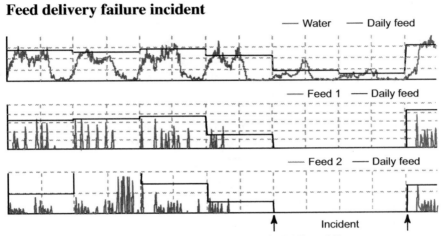

Figure 6.8 A serious incident involving feed delivery failure

Figure 6.8 is a print out from Barn Report which logged a serious incident when feed augers failed to function for several days. The incident arose during a weekend. Water intake was severely disrupted even though room temperature reached almost 32 C (90F) by Sunday. The reason for this mishap was that the feed delivery system actually failed on Friday morning and soon after the feed hoppers had been eaten empty. When the feed supply was restored after the weekend, feed and water intake increased but the original levels were not achieved for several days.

Things can only get worse!

When *ad-lib* hoppers become empty pigs are not slow to bring this to the attention of those who care for them. However, if pigs miss lunch they do

not have two dinners to redress the balance. If feed becomes unavailable to
a pig that was actively seeking it, this must be regarded as a lost opportunity
that can never be retrieved.

Scale of operation brings with it an increased dependence on automation.
Feed delivery systems tend to be semi-automatic, *i.e.* manually triggered but
stopping without human interference when the hopper is full. Alternatively,
they are fully automatic, *i.e.* they run as and when required. Automation
sometimes goes wrong. If a pig keeper discovers a somewhat depleted
feed hopper which has not been topped-up automatically, the chances are
the dominant pigs have already monopolised the hopper's feeding spaces
at the expense of the shy feeders. If a feed hopper becomes completely
empty, not only is there a productivity loss but the likelihood is that pigs
would become aggressive and outbreaks of tail biting become more likely.
Data logging presents a great opportunity to ascertain whether automated
feeding systems are 'delivering the goods' as intended.

Figure 6.9 shows a comparison of auger operation on a new seven room
finishing site over a 30 month period. It was set up to run as many times a
day as was needed to keep the hoppers full.

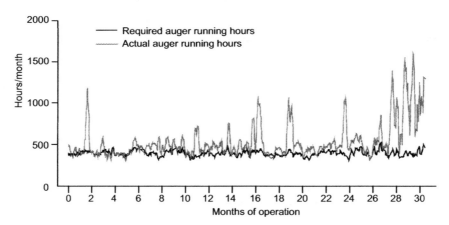

Figure 6.9 Progressive efficiency losses within an automated feeding system

Each of the seven hoppers were required to run for almost 2 hours per day,
i.e. a total running time for all hoppers of around 400 hours per month.
This is depicted by the bold line on the graph which shows a rolling average
of how much the augers should be running. The small degree of variation
reflects the fact that the required running time is dominated by the age and

different needs of pigs in the different buildings. The red line shows how long the seven hoppers were actually running over the monitoring period.

As expected at the outset, the two lines are fairly close together. This arises because the augers were operating as required, *i.e.* they ran for as long as was necessary to replenish the feed as it was used. The occasional blips in the line reflect incidents such as feed bridging within the bulk storage bin. This is a common problem on many units and in this instance arose within the first month after the new building and feed system were commissioned. After a few months, the line blips become more frequent and they are spread over a longer time interval. In other words, although in the early days of operation feed delivery was reasonably reliable, as time progressed there was a marked deterioration in the system and to deliver the same goods, the augers had to be used for longer periods.

In most instances, clandestine deterioration of this order would not be noticed by those operating the system. A degree of topping-up takes place, but in the main, this remains unseen. It is reasonable to assume that on occasions some pigs would not have received the food they were required to consume and this was not observed.

This is yet another instance of data-logging being used to confirm all is well or to give unit managers an early indication when all is not well. An empty feed hopper certainly alerts the stock-keeper to the fact that all is not well but it provides no clues as to the duration of this shortcoming and its true cost.

Water feed intake on a contract finishing system

The following case study relates to a situation in which a contract finisher regularly struggled to achieve acceptable performance. The climatic environment was checked and found to be in good order but the pigs failed to perform despite apparently being in good health. Whenever feed hoppers were checked, they were found to be full.

The Barn Report data summarised in Figure 6.10 was collected over an eight day period and refers to water and feed intake in a particular building. The period of monitoring coincided with an episode of hot summer weather when daytime ambient temperature often peaked at 30°C (86°F). The downward steps on the lighter line indicate that water intake fell when augers failed to deliver feed and pigs stopped eating. The pigs were approaching slaughter weight and the graphs indicated a close relationship between eating and drinking. Even though temperature levels were high, water intake was lower than expected; this arose because the high ambient temperature had suppressed interest in feeding. The underlying message is that water uptake is more closely linked with feed intake rather than temperature *per se*.

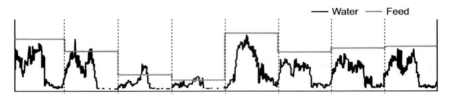

Figure 6.10 Water and feed intake on a contract pig finishing system

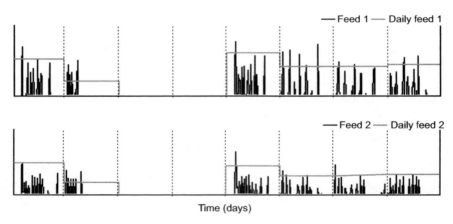

Time (days)

Figure 6.11 Feed delivery from specific augers

Figure 6.11 refers to two different augers within the same system and which have been labelled as 'Feed 1' and 'Feed 2'. The boldly printed spikes depict auger runs for the two hoppers and the lighter lines show the total daily auger run times. Pigs failed to receive any food for three days. The associated drop in water intake shown in Figure 6.10 represents a fall of 78.6%. However, when feed delivery was restored, water consumption rapidly increased.

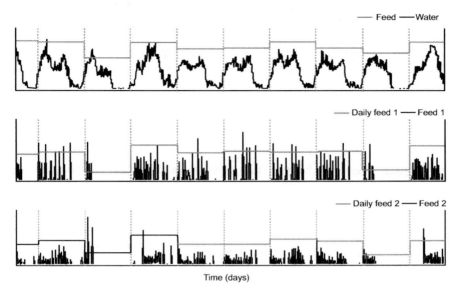

Figure 6.12 Earlier feed delivery problems on automated systems

When this data logged information was first observed, it seemed reasonable to assume that feed delivery failures had been isolated incidents. Figure 6.12 demonstrates that this was far from the reality. Since the data-logger was already in place, it was possible to appraise historical records. The data shown in Figure 6.12 was collected two weeks before that in Figures 6.10 and 6.11. Two significant 'feed out' situations are apparent and it is assumed that these arose because of feed bridging. Although not shown on the graph, both these incidents arose around midday and the augers were unable to deliver feed before 7.30 am the next day. Since the feed very likely ran out overnight, the consequences would have been largely unseen. Contract finishing depends on the hiring of suitable buildings and pigs are often cared for by people whose principal focus and skills are land based rather than pig based. If, in this installation, the contractor and contractee had together been using data-logging as a daily management aid, the problem would have been spotted earlier, efficiency would have been improved and bonus payments would, very likely, have accrued.

'Dribbling' and 'Sticking' – unseen threats to water supply

Besides shortcomings in feed delivery systems, often water distribution is compromised because of unseen faults within the plumbing system. On many pig units water supply from a cistern or header tank is controlled by a well hidden float-valve, *i.e.* a ballcock. The float valve automatically opens to facilitate water flow when the water level drops below a certain value. Provided this threshold capacity remains available, the float valve closes and this inhibits water flow. The two most common faults are 'dribbling' and 'sticking'. When dribbling takes place, the ballcock fails to shut off, whereas when it sticks, the valve remains closed and water flow is inhibited

Figure 6.13 describes a situation on a pig unit where the water flow rate was generally not hindered by dribbling or sticking within the header tank.

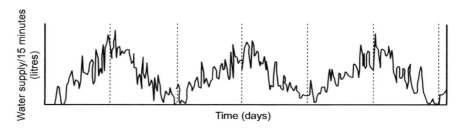

Figure 6.13 A typical water logging trace

The chart shows the water delivery pattern in a pig building over a three day period. The vertical axis refers to water flow rate whilst the horizontal axis refers to time. Figure 6.13 shows that water kept flowing throughout almost the whole of the recording period. The minimum delivery rate was around 0.5 litres/15 minutes (0.28 pints/15 minutes). In effect, after 0.5 litres (0.28 pints) is removed from the header tank, the valve on the ballcock opens and tops up the water level. In situations represented by the peaks *i.e.* at the highest water flow rates, the header tank will have opened and closed many times in any 15 minute recording period. In effect in the situation recorded, the valve will very likely have opened between 300 and 500 times per day; in a full year this would amount to something approaching 100,000 to 200,000 times. This degree of use is at least ten times the demand that would be typical for heavy domestic or industrial water supply systems. The implication is that wear and tear on a pig unit ballcock system is such that valve seats very likely would need replacing at least annually.

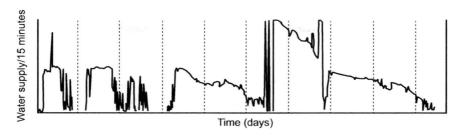

Figure 6.14 A serious problem within the water supply system

Not all systems work as well as that described in the foregoing case study. Figure 6.14 demonstrates what can happen if maintenance to the plumbing system is inadequate. The flow rate was erratic. When the valve opened, there was a surge of water and it gushed through the pipeline at such a rate that much of it was lost through the slatted floor and produced an inconveniently dilute slurry.

Figure 6.15 shows a situation in which there were prolonged periods with a low flow rate of water.

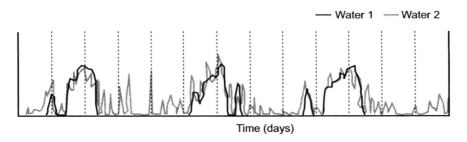

Figure 6.15 A problem with continuously dribbling water

The data refer to a three day monitoring period involving two header tanks (Water 1 and Water 2). Water 1 has a problem because there is virtually no water removal at night despite some predictable peaks of water flow rate being achieved during the day. On the graph shown in Figure 6.15, the darker line represents the problematic Water 1 tank. A marked feature of the trace is the total absence of the darker line for long periods at night. On the other hand, the lighter spiky trace (Water 2) provides a more uniform water usage pattern much nearer the requirement of the pigs.

The reason for the problem in the header tank Water 1 is that water was continuously dribbling from the ballcock valve. However, its flow rate was so slow that it did not register on the water meter. It ran continuously and over-filled the tank. Eventually the surplus stored water would be consumed and this would result in the valve operating at full flow rate to allow the tank to refill. The two header tanks were sited within the same room and pig behaviour suggested that all pigs supplied from the header tanks were getting sufficient water. However, the overall un-metered water dribbling through the defective system resulted in 10-30% extra demand for water. This is not a smart way of managing a scarce resource.

7

THE CONSEQUENCES OF EXCESSIVE TEMPERATURE BUILD-UP

In temperate zones, thermostatically controlled ventilation systems aim to maintain a constant temperature usually in the 15-30°C (59-86°F) range depending on the age of the pig. If the ambient temperature exceeds that of the target room temperature, the ventilation system cannot keep the room temperature close to the target. Typically, the best outcome would be to keep room temperature no more than about 3°C (37.4°F) hotter than the outside temperature when the room is stocked and the ventilation system is working flat-out. In other words, if the target room temperature is 24°C (75.2°F) in a fully stocked finishing house, operating at maximum ventilation rate, the temperature would be likely to reach 27°C (80.6°F) and there would be no risk of the pigs coming to immediate harm since the available ventilation would allow them to lose excess body heat, however, feed intake would very likely be impaired and the pigs would show signs of discomfort. Nevertheless, if the room temperature soared much higher, the consequences could be very serious. This could arise because of a further increase in the ambient temperature, the consequences of over-stocking or failure of some or all of the ventilation system. In order to safeguard the welfare of the pigs, comply with regulations or conditions of insurance, alarm systems are usually fitted to alert operators when to intervene. These alarms are generally triggered by excessive temperature rise, although factors such as lack of oxygen, excessive build-up of carbon dioxide or the build-up of toxic gases from slurry could each in themselves be lethal. Alarms tend to be referred to as 'over temperature alarms'. This is a misnomer since it tends to down-play the earlier mentioned potentially lethal factors. The real purpose of an alarm is to indicate that there are serious shortcomings in the pig environment; the incidence of excessive temperature build-up is simply used as the messenger of this bad news. In other words, if temperature is used as the messenger, by the time the building operator is alerted or fail-safe equipment is activated, the welfare and productivity of the housed pigs could well have been compromised. This tendency is exacerbated by the practice of simply setting the alarm trigger to a higher temperature than that normally expected. Typically, alarm temperatures are set around 30-35°C (86°-95°F). There is little scientific basis for this and practical considerations such as the avoidance of 'false' alarms tend to dominate.

There has been little research undertaken on this key aspect of pig welfare and production efficiency. Reported research tends to focus on the impact on the pigs during the first 20 minutes after the alarm is activated. With little justification, the assumption is made that the temperature rise would remain constant. Whereas globally millions of pigs are at risk of dying because of ventilation failure, the number actually that do die is very low. Apart from honouring welfare responsibilities, pig farmers cannot afford to bear the cost of high mortalities. When pigs do die after the build-up of excessively high temperatures, mortalities tend to be high. However, throughout the global pig industry, the frequency of 'near-misses' is much more widespread. There is an unqualified acceptance that if pigs have not died, their welfare has not been compromised and any production loss has been transient and insignificant. There is no scientific basis for this mindset.

Excessive temperature build-up and ventilation failure alarms

Data from actual incidents are sparse and so any information that is available is worthy of close scrutiny. The following paragraphs review two such incidents where prolonged ventilation failure arose on commercial farms. It is only possible to review the likely impact of these mishaps because temperature logging equipment was routinely used on these farms

As illustrated earlier, controlled environment buildings need a large *temperature lift* potential in order to achieve desired temperatures; for example, to achieve 20°C (68°F) inside, the temperature lift potential must be at least 25°C (77°F) when it is -5°C (23°F) outside. Controlled ventilation removes the excess heat. If ventilation fails, less heat is removed, so room temperature rises. Increased temperature can, therefore, be a useful indication of failure. With no or insufficient ventilation, pigs may die because of excessive temperature, as a consequence of suffocation arising from too much carbon dioxide and/or too little oxygen, toxic gases from slurry - or perhaps a combination of any or all of these.

In some countries, including the UK, compliance with welfare regulations necessitates the installation and regular testing of ventilation failure alarms.

In other countries, alarms are not required by law, although many producers have them, either as a management tool, or because of an insurance policy requirement. It is by no means clear whether the installation of an alarm system actually has a positive impact on the incidence of ventilation failure or any resultant stress to pigs. Since temperature is inclined to rise in the event of ventilation failure and excess temperature is a likely cause of death, high temperature alarm is the most common method of detecting ventilation failure.

High temperature is not itself the failure, but rather a *symptom* of ventilation failure. High temperature alarms are, therefore, a common way to *detect* ventilation failure. Whilst the safety of pigs is often placed in the hands of high temperature alarms, a major weakness of such a system is that setting these alarms is in the hands of the human operators. Consequently, the level of understanding - and the due diligence - of the human operators is paramount.

As with any other type of automation, it is only as good as the way it is used because of its reliance on human understanding. Mistakes are more likely to be made by untrained operators who lack the appropriate understanding. This is particularly so when alarms are triggered "out of hours" because invariably someone is subjected to a degree of inconvenience whether justified or otherwise.

In practice, understanding of the role, function and effective operation of ventilation failure alarms tends to be lacking. One of the reasons for this is that there is relatively little objective information on what actually happens when ventilation fails.

Ventilation failure incidents have been little investigated; even when investigated, there is often little hard evidence, and so the focus tends to be establishing fault or liability rather than determining exactly what happened.

Ventilation failure incident in eight farrowing rooms

The incident arose in a group of eight farrowing rooms within a single building. Air entered the building via barometric air inlets. The mishap occurred at around midnight, on a mild July night when ambient temperature was around 14°C (57.2°F), the mains supply to the whole building was tripped out by an RCD, due to an electrical fault. This disconnected power to all circuits including fans, heaters, lighting and controllers.

As it happened, temperature logging was already underway. Every 15 minutes temperatures were being recorded by a Dicam® logging system with a sensitivity around ±0.3°C (32.5°F). Back-up batteries in controllers provided temporary monitoring for five to eight hours after the mains loss.

Ambient wind speed was around 2.7m/sec (6 mph) but data logging indicated little impact from the wind since the ventilation system was well baffled.

Figures 7.1 and 7.2 show temperatures in the eight farrowing rooms following the mains loss. The steady horizontal line (Fig. 7.1) depicts ambient temperature.

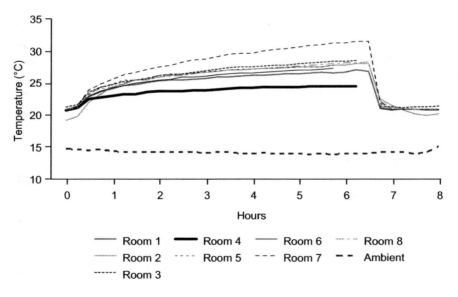

Figure 7.1 A ventilation failure incident in farrowing rooms

The loss of mains electricity occurred just after the start of the temperature recording chart shown, at which point there was a sudden rise in temperature of 2 - 3°C (6°F) in each room.

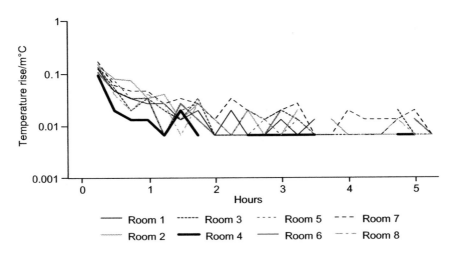

Figure 7.2 Rate of temperature rise

The starting temperature in Room 2 was a little lower than those in the other rooms which were around 21°C (69.8°F). However, after the mains failure the temperature lift in the seven occupied rooms varied somewhat. Room 4 air temperature increased to 24.5°C (76.1°F) but in Room 7 the piglets were heavier and so had greater heat output. In this room, air temperature actually reached 32°C (89.6°F) after nearly seven hours.

Temperature rise (Figure 7.2), varied from room to room since each room housed sows at a different stage of lactation.. Room 7 had the oldest litters, and therefore the greatest temperature rise. Temperature rose relatively quickly at first - 0.1 to 0.15°C (0.2 - 0.3°F) per minute but this sharp rise only persisted for 30 to 60 minutes, then it slowed down. Thereafter, the rate of temperature increase fell to only 0.007 to 0.015°C per minute (around 32.03°F per minute).

Temperature lift in the absence of ventilation was clearly asymptotic (Figure 7.1). That is, it increased towards a new, higher, temperature - but the closer it approached this point, the slower the rise became. This is not what most people would have expected. If the ventilation were switched off and the temperature rose 3°C (5°F) in 20 minutes, the expectation would be for it to be 6°C (10°F) higher in 40 minutes, 9°C (16°F) in 60 minutes, and so on. The perception is that, whatever trigger temperature has been set, it will be reached sooner or later. This, however, does not happen in practice.

This asymptotic characteristic arises for two main reasons. The first is concerned with basic physics. As temperature rises, the difference between inside and outside increases, and so more and more heat is lost to the outside, leaving less to cause further temperature rise. The second is that the pigs are not a 'simple' heat source – they are, however, 'a quasi-constant temperature source'. As room temperature rises, the animals find it more and more difficult to dissipate heat into the environment - a fact which causes a rise in body temperature, and ultimately death.

The important implication of this is that to have any real hope of success, high temperature alarms must trigger soon after the failure itself. If they are not set close to the normal operating temperature - so they trigger during the initial phase of temperature rise - they may take a very long time to trigger, or not trigger at all. Therefore in situations where electrical power fails, 'time to trigger' is crucial; in the very worst situation it could mean the difference between pigs living and dying.

Table 7.1 indicates the impact of 'time to trigger' and demonstrates that small differences in a high temperature trigger point would have a large effect.

Table 7.1 The impact of time to trigger high temperature warning

| Alarm trigger point | | Time taken to exceed |
°C	°F	trigger point (hours)
24	75.2	1.0
25	77.0	2.0
26	78.8	4.0
27		Not exceeded

Using Room 1 as an example, Table 7.1 indicates how long it would have taken before alarms were raised at different temperatures for the alarm trigger point. Obviously, the higher the trigger point, the longer it takes before there is any likelihood of remedial action. If the trigger point in Room 1 had been set at 27°C (80.6°F) it would not have been exceeded until at least four hours after the mains failure. Referring back to Figure 7.1, it can be seen that in Room 7 the temperature eventually exceeded 30°C (86°F) after four hours. Put another way, had the temperature trigger been 30°C (86°F), it would only have been activated in Room 7 in the case study presented, assuming the device was accurate.

If the ambient temperature had been lower on that July night, it would have taken much longer for the over temperature trigger to be activated. As it happened, no pigs died, but given the build-up in room temperature and the delay of automatic remedial action, the welfare of the housed pigs would have been compromised. It seems that the mindset of pig unit operators has been dominated by the need to avoid ultimate disasters during the event of a power failure. The cost of this delayed safeguard is the likelihood that pigs would be subjected to a metabolic crisis long before disaster strikes.

In this particular incident, the alarm was triggered by the general mains failure, and an operative arrived shortly thereafter. However, the operator did not know what to do, failed to spot the tripped RCD, failed to check the pigs and did not think of leaving the doors open. This is a 'sharp-end' example of an investment in sophisticated equipment being ineffective because of inadequate investment in staff training.

Ventilation failure incident in a dry sow house

This case study describes an electrical failure with serious consequences in a large dry sow and service house in a hot climate. Ventilation failure arose because a circuit breaker was accidentally switched off during early afternoon, *i.e.* human error. Unfortunately the problem was not discovered and remedial action undertaken for some 16 hours when staff first returned to the site the next morning. The local climate was such that evaporative cooling had been installed in the building, so at the start of this serious incident, the room temperature was actually lower than ambient. (Evaporative coolers are wetted plates in the air inlets. Water evaporation reduces the dry bulb temperature of the incoming air towards the dew point temperature so air temperature is lower than outside, as long as the ventilation and water pump are working properly.) Even so, on extreme occasions room temperatures as high has 33.5°C (92.3°F) had been recorded in this building despite assistance from reliable fully functional ventilation and evaporative cooling equipment. Sows actually died as a result of the incident described in this case study. Furthermore, there were many resultant abortions and so in addition to the welfare impact, significant production losses would have arisen.

Figure 7.3. shows temperatures over a 16 hour period following a loss of ventilation. In this instance, the initial temperature inside the house was lower than outside - due to the use of evaporative coolers.

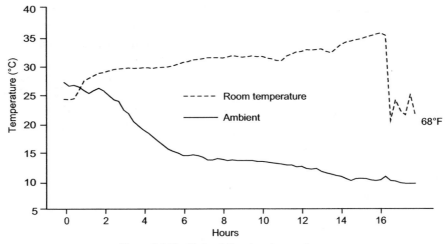

Figure 7.3 Ventilation failure in a dry sow house

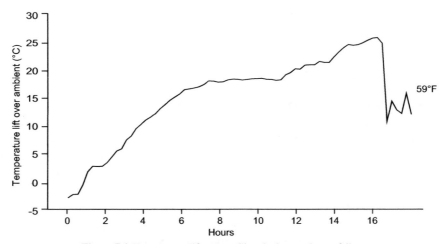

Figure 7.4 Temperature lift over ambient in dry sow house failure

As before, there was an initial rise of a few degrees - and thereafter temperature crawled slowly upwards , but on occasions there were temperature falls. This probably arose because changes in wind direction and air speed affected open air inlets in the building. Furthermore, the incident was an overnight event and arose during a period of falling ambient temperature. A very significant factor in the situation described was the outside temperature. Although the house temperature continued to rise *relative* to outside (see Figure 7.4), it was climbing only slowly in absolute terms.

It can be seen from Figure 7.3 that soon after the incident occurred, ambient temperature was falling as evening approached. Nevertheless the number and high body weight of the sows and boars brought about a continued rate of rise around 0.05°C/minute (32.09°F/minute) compared to the ambient temperature, the actual rate of rise was only around 0.01°C/minute (32.02°F/minute).

After 16 hours, room temperature reached 35.5°C (96°F). However, the high temperature alarm never actually triggered, even though it was 27°C (81°F) at the start of the incident. This is because the high temperature alarm trigger was set to 36°C (97°F).

As in the previous case study, it is possible to pinpoint temperature trigger times at various trigger settings. This is shown in Table 7.2.

Table 7.2 The impact of time to trigger high temperature warning

| Alarm trigger point | | Time taken to exceed |
°C	°F	trigger point (hours)
27	80.6	<1.0
29	84.2	2.5
31	87.8	7.0
33	91.4	14.0
35	95.0	15.5

Had the trigger point been 33°C (91.4°F) it would have taken more than half a day before remedial action would have been effective. Temperature simply measures 'how hot' it is within a particular situation, not 'how suitable' that situation might be.

This incident was caused by *human error*, not electrical fault. The circuit breaker for the feed system was next to the circuit breaker for the fans. On this farm, the feeding system was switched off at night. On this occasion, the fan circuit was switched off by mistake. The mains failure alarm system was powered from a separate circuit breaker.

This illustrates a second general point. Pigs are left alone for most of the time, often for 16 hours or more during the night when temperatures are typically falling. High temperature triggers set for daytime operation may simply not have any impact at all during the night.

Control system failure in a farrowing room

Figure 7.5 shows temperature measured in a farrowing room - one of eight - over a weekend *i.e.* Friday evening through to Sunday. It was hot weather - on Saturday afternoon, outside temperature reached 31°C (88°F). In this building, controls were older individual control units, whilst conversely, alarm and data logging were provided by an up-to-date network system. Since the room had evaporative coolers, inside temperatures were lower than outside.

At around 8 pm on the second day, a severe thunderstorm passed through the locality and this was reflected in a sharp drop in the outside temperature shown in Figure 7.5. Six of the rooms carried on working normally, two did not and one of these is featured in this example.

The temperature rose quickly in the first hour; 5°C (9°F), but in the next hour the rise was only about 1°C (2°F) and in the third hour only about 0.5°C (1°F). By 1 am, 5 hours after the incident, - it had eventually reached 34°C (93°F).

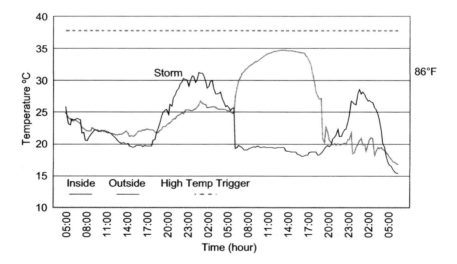

Figure 7.5 Control system failure in farrowing room

The high temperature alarm was set at 38°C (100°F). Clearly, it was never going to reach that point. One might well ask why it was set so high, given that with ventilation and evaporative cooling functioning normally, the highest temperature that had been reached in any of the rooms in previous months was 29°C (84°F) when it was 35°C (95°F) outside.

At what point, exactly, animals started to die is not clear. Possibly around 4 am on Sunday morning, when temperature lift stopped rising.

People problems or equipment failure problems?

In the first incident, a simple electrical fault led to a loss of mains, which triggered mains failure alarms. The operator attended, but didn't know what to do. The second incident was caused by human error in switching off the wrong circuit. The third was an actual controller breakdown, caused by an electrical storm.

In all three cases, high temperature alarms - which were fully functional - were not triggered because they were set too high. In the second and third cases, they were set so as to allow for high outside temperatures, even though the evaporative cooling kept inside temperatures lower than outside.

In all these incidents, suspicion was pointed at controls and alarms but in all three cases, the "human factor" was largely if not entirely the issue. Alarms were functioning correctly, but they were set so as to positively avoid alarming, rather than detect potential problems.

There are, then very good reasons for third party monitoring of pig farms using broadband and related technology. If data and readings were available elsewhere than on the farm, it would make it possible to use more advanced techniques and software to determine the best course of action in any given circumstances. This could apply not just to acute alarms - where pigs are at immediate risk of harm – but to longer term anomalies.

However, before such concepts can become a reality, the pig industry must be receptive to radical new thinking. Not least, it means changing the mindset from thinking of short term 'payback' to one of commitment to developing, expanding and improving production technology to achieve medium and long term goals.

Limiting the impact of temperature build-up

Although there were shortcomings in staff training and management protocols, the three incidents reviewed arose because inappropriate alarm trigger points had been set. On most pig units, alarm systems are installed primarily to prevent death of pigs following power failure. Whereas death is absolute, temporary production losses arising because of the unsuitability of the pigs' environment are imprecise. They are not measured so their economic impact is unknown. Under commercial farming conditions, operators are generally therefore unable to quantify any cost benefit that might arise as a result of installing more sophisticated alarm devices such as gas detection equipment, bearing in mind suffocation rather than temperature *per se* is the problem. Detecting ventilation failure based on a fixed high temperature trigger point is a questionable practice. Assuming that any particular temperature will be reached 'sooner or later' is too imprecise. Using an *absolute* value for the temperature trigger does not indicate that the ventilation is no longer functioning or whether the pigs are stressed.

It is common practice for pigs to be left unchecked by humans for 12-18 hours. If power failure arises during this crucial interval it is highly likely that although pigs might not die, the absence of ventilation will impair their well-being and productivity. In the absence of detailed research, pinpointing more meaningful high temperature trigger points is difficult. However, the second case study reviewed indicated that the triggering point was activated far too late. How might this be remedied given the reluctance to invest in more sophisticated triggering devices?

When ventilation fails and temperature rises, *temperature lift* over *ambient* results, rather than an *absolute* temperature. The two case studies indicate that the largest part of the temperature rise occurs during the initial stages. Around two thirds of the temperature lift that might arise within four hours actually arose within the first 30 minutes. Hence there is a strong argument for the trigger temperature to be activated shortly after increased room temperature becomes a physical reality.

In individual pig buildings it is worth testing the impact of ventilation failure. If ventilation is switched off during mild or cool ambient temperatures, the resultant room temperature should be recorded and then related to the ambient temperature. This temperature lift could then be used as the basis for setting the high temperature trigger and automatically taking account of an 'operating margin' above *set temperature*, or above *ambient temperature*.

In effect, room temperature could be allowed to increase, *e.g.* 5°C (41°F) above the set temperature or 5°C (41°F) above ambient when ambient exceeds room temperature. This automatically increases the trigger point when the ambient temperature is higher and reduces it again when it is cooler. In this way the high temperature point is triggered at a more appropriate point and the probability of false activation is decreased.

A new sense of direction

Whilst there are clear limitations associated with the technique of detecting ventilation faults and problems by means of temperature, this is not to suggest abandoning or avoiding the technique. In a temperature-based ventilation system, an error in temperature achieved is an indication of a potential problem that should be addressed.

One way to improve high temperature alarms is to use ambient over-temperature compensation. Modern software-based temperature alarms have a facility, or can have one added to measure and compensate for elevated outside temperatures. This raises thresholds automatically when it is warmer outside but - crucially - lowers them when ambient temperatures fall and buildings can achieve normal targets again. Thresholds can be set closer to normal operating temperatures so that they trigger during the initial temperature rise following a ventilation failure, but are not triggered by increases in ambient temperature during warmer weather.

Setting temperature thresholds nearer the recommended room temperature increases the likelihood of "false positives". The tighter they are set, the more likely they may trigger even if equipment is working properly. By contrast, setting margins wider means false positives are less likely, but makes it more likely that genuine problems will be missed. Even when they are detected - eventually - the suffering and impairment to growth are likely to be greater, the longer detection takes.

From a financial perspective, it is better to accept a higher level of 'false positives' than like many, deliberately set alarm triggers so that they avoid them. If it costs, *e.g.*, £20 ($36) to attend an alarm, and the cost in lost growth of an unattended failure would have been £200 ($360), up to 9 false positives for every real positive is advantageous. If a missed alarm cost

£5000 ($9,000) in dead animals, distress to staff and the risk of criminal proceedings, then working on a 100 to 1 probability would make good business sense.

An important shift in emphasis then is to train staff to 'love their alarms' - to treat them as a friend, rather than an irritating enemy who drags them out of bed unnecessarily. This can be a difficult task, but it may be more achievable if staff were generously recompensed for effectively managing alarm systems by rewarding diligence - for every call out, false or otherwise. Alarms may well be regarded as devices that indicate a problem, but maybe they should also be regarded as devices that should be regularly checked to confirm normality.

8

I.T. – THE GLOBAL DRIVER OF FUTURE PIG PRODUCTION

Those committed to a profitable future in an increasingly global pig industry do not have the option to stand and watch whilst others progress. The risk of the traditional pig industry becoming a victim of 'technological leap-frogging' by countries wishing to intensify production has already been highlighted. Pig meat is the most widely consumed meat in the world and consumption trends are rising; these are statistical realities.

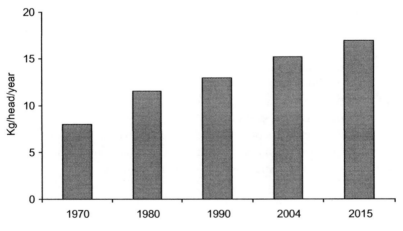

Figure 8.1 Pigmeat consumption 1970 to 2015

Based on figures extracted from the FAO database, Roppa (2004) suggests that annual global pig meat consumption figures will be around 17.5kg (39 lb)/head/year by 2015 (Figure 8.1). He predicts that associated with this growth there will be a doubling of current sow numbers from 8.2 million to 16.3 million by 2015. Furthermore, much of this growth will arise in the less developed countries; Brazil, Russia, India and China are likely to be major players. Meanwhile, coping with cost and regulatory burdens will be a continuing feature of pig farming in developed countries. Consumers of pork in these countries have demanded a high degree of food safety and traceability and changing the source of supply is unlikely to change these expectations. Less developed countries expanding their pig industries will therefore maximise their advantages of climate and their abundance of land and availability of water. Lower labour costs will also be an important feature of their production systems. Increased use of production technology will ensure that they too produce high quality pork which is safe to eat and is health assured. Consumers will continue to demand farm to fork assurance which embraces traceability, quality, welfare considerations and compliance with government regulations within a sustainable production environment. I.T. will, therefore, play a major role in helping meet these challenging objectives since market forces will demand it. This has already happened within the global broiler industry in that countries once regarded as less developed, because they carried no historical baggage, have been able to make themselves major poultry meat suppliers to discerning consumers in distant lands. Although established pig producing countries will be likely to concentrate on value-added production, if they are to survive within a competitive marketplace, they will have to operate under the same 'club rules'.

Some people, because of ethical considerations, are not comfortable with the concept of the industrialization of agriculture. However, 'biological manufacturing', will become widespread with food manufacturers competing within their specific food chain. Given the predicted increased global demand for pigmeat products, pig production does not have the option of becoming a sunset industry. Crabtree (2006) has summarised the likely key drivers of the future increasingly global pig industry.

- Pork is the global meat of choice and will continue to be so.

- Pig production will shift from developed to developing markets.

- Full production integration will take place recognizing the need for process control and whole chain monitoring.

- Food companies will become dominant as food chain versus food chain competition evolves.

- Food production will have to take a more holistic approach successfully integrating food quality, competitive pricing, being consumer responsive, traceability, security from food terrorism, environmental sustainability and ethical responsibility.

- A massive challenge that quite obviously will need all the help it can get from innovative, flexible and open information systems.

Exploiting the benefits of I.T.

The pig industry is failing to make the most of I.T. know-how which is already widely used in manufacturing industries, particularly where consistency and quality control are paramount. Independent pig recording systems suggest that 'hit and miss' management prevails on many UK pig units and is manifested in the wide variation of results achieved on commercial pig farms. The British Pig Executive Yearbook for 2007 indicates 11% faster growth rates on 'Top 10%' recorded finishing herds compared to 'Average' herds. (Table 8.1)

Table 8.1 Overall feeding herd results, year ended Sept 2006

	Average	*Top Third*	*Top 10%*
Herd Structure			
Average No. of pigs	1,992	2,493	3,314
Pig performance			
Weight of pigs at start (kg)	27.2	33.5	40.6
Weight of pigs produced (kg)	98.2	102.0	103.5
Mortality (%)	5.6	4.9	5.1
Feed conversion ratio	2.75:1	2.84:1	2.82:1
Daily gain (g)	655	706	727

Source: BPEX Pig Yearbook 2007
(BPEX 2007)

These results imply that either existing monitoring systems are inadequate or irrelevant or that those that are in place are not being used advantageously. Industrialists would say that existing 'pig production plant' monitoring protocols are inadequate. I.T. must be increasingly used to ensure that there is more on-going attention to detail and regular analysis and modification of the pig environment so that target performance is consistently achieved. Put another way, when science indicates that changes are needed within a building, such changes should be automatically implemented before sub-optimal performance takes hold.

When pig farmers first used computers, hardware costs were reduced by sharing them with others. They subscribed to a bureau system, *i.e.* paid money so that their businesses could benefit from the latest technology. Low cost computers with massive capacity are now directly available to the business world. Meanwhile, people have become expensive along with travel and on-farm biosecurity. Progressive pig farmers are therefore, more prepared to buy time and expertise by investing in software development and knowledge transfer. The pioneers of computerised pig recording systems acknowledge that they had masses of potentially informative data, much of which was never analysed, so it did not significantly contribute to the development of their pig businesses. They rectified this situation by purchasing I.T. expertise which was readily available from established technologies which were already in widespread use in other industries.

Depending on the size of the pig unit, new methods of harnessing I.T. know-how in relation to the pig environment will now have to be engaged. Large scale producers might well incorporate in-house bespoke information management systems or depend on out-sourcing. Smaller pig enterprises where long-term capital investment is less affordable will be more comfortable with pre-budgeted monthly payments into a specialist bureau system. In other words, the full value of sophisticated hardware will be realized via developing an on-going relationship with the supplier of that hardware. The mindset of the pig farmer will have to change in that there must be recognition of the need to pay for this specialist knowledge and expertise which will drive the modern industry.

Those who supply technology to low volume specialist markets such as the pig industry are often subjected to heavy unsustainable technical demands from the end user whose main focus is inevitably on the pigs rather than the environment around them. Conversely, those manufacturers in other industries who supply the mass market attempt to design their way out of trouble by making their products user-friendly and unlikely to generate any demand for regular contact between supplier and end user. Specialist markets will, however, continue to need bespoke 'proactive technical support' and will buy-in expertise via 'actionable recommendations'. This approach will enable pig farmers to introduce necessary changes within the pig environment, leaving themselves more time to do what they do best with enhanced job satisfaction arising from the resultant increase in technical efficiency.

Masses of inaccessible, undecipherable data will not help boost the efficiency of modern pig farming. However, remote automatic processing of that data and the provision of intelligible, actionable recommendations will help overcome the end-user's lack of time and skills shortage. Pig management cannot be improved unless the people managing pigs understand their environment needs and provide them at all times. Suppliers of monitoring equipment should, therefore, concentrate their efforts on sharing their specialist knowledge with those who manage the pigs. Some might argue that computerised remote management is unethical. However, if the outcome is that the welfare of the pigs is improved, such arguments bear little weight.

Learning from other industries

As yet few pig farmers have a permanent direct link between their environment monitoring devices and the Internet. In this respect the pig industry is lagging behind other industries outside of agriculture. Telemetry is in widespread use globally. It involves automated machine to machine communication, often referred to as 'M2M technology'. It started way back in the US Apollo space missions and was then very costly. The same technology has become low cost and is widely used in the form of SIM card devices. It has been estimated that within Europe alone, some 13 billion devices have the potential to communicate directly with each other without human intervention. These devices range from vending machines and parking meters to fire alarms and photocopiers. M2M technology is not restricted by geographical boundaries and has the ability to inform and assist lone workers in remote situations.

The potential of M2M is mind-bending. Not only does it benefit the end user but it also helps the manufacturer have a better understanding of the potential and limitations of the 'gadgetry' supplied. Device networking enables, *e.g.* the manufacturers of washing machines, to be informed immediately if a breakdown arises. It can be used as a means of pro-actively informing the consumer that there has been a breakdown and that immediate service is underway. If washing machine manufacturers are able to use their connected products to generate customer service relationships, why cannot the pig industry adopt the same technology? Manufacturers of pig environment monitoring equipment could use device-networking technology which would take the hassle out of hard-pressed pig unit managers needing to make subjective decisions.

This is not 'pig pie in the sky'. Consider how the Internet already connects millions of people worldwide. Within industry and in domestic situations there are millions of devices which could be connected to the Internet and facilitate automatic global communication, data collection and device control. The modern pig industry must be pro-active in embracing this new technology and become part of the inflection point which will herald the next stage in Internet usage. When referring to the coverage of machine to machine communications, I.T. specialists speak of the 'Pervasive Internet' which will dominate data handling and interpretation across a range of global industries. The concept is outlined in Figure 8.2. (Comtech Ltd 2006).

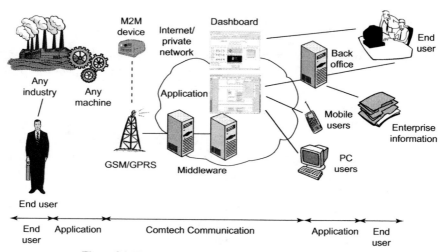

Figure 8.2 The way ahead: machine to machine communication

Whilst pig people might be daunted by such technology, understanding how it works is unimportant. Application of this technology will be the key issue. Imagine running a pig building with monitoring devices permanently on line, the potential is amazing. Parameters such as weather, feed, water, house temperature, dust, bug counts, cough counts and even pig behaviour not only could be permanently monitored but, by being connected to the appropriate engine of analysis, on-going interpretation will be possible.

Pig producers will have to become more integrated within their particular supply chain and as a consequence will benefit from the use of networked 'embedded intelligence'. This will become the driver of quality control, consistency and economy of production. Pork chains will increasingly reflect product differentiation and I.T. devices installed within pig buildings will reflect this need for differentiation.

The aggressiveness of the pig environment is such that electronic devices operating within the same hostile air space as pigs have suffered a difficult gestation, but the associated difficulties have been largely overcome. Early adopters of the Internet struggled with wires and connectors but now enjoy the luxury of reliable wireless connectivity. Bad experiences with wiring which is always prone to vermin attack have been one reason why the pig industry has been slow to install wired monitoring devices within pig buildings. The pig farmer of the future will not only use electronic devices which automatically monitor and modify the environment, but they will also reap the benefits of proven wireless connectivity.

REFERENCES

BPEX (2007) British Pig Executive, Pig Yearbook 2007, 39-55

Comtech Ltd (2006) www.comtech2m.com

Crabtree, H.G. (2006) Can the promise of I.T. become a reality in pig production? The Royal Agricultural Club and Nat West 100 Club Annual Fellowship in Pig Research: Report No. 5

Defra (2003) Code of Recommendations for the Welfare of Livestock: Pigs

Roppa, L (2005) Global Pig Meat Production – 2005 Banff Pork Seminar

Smith, P., Crabtree, H.G. (2005) Pig Environment Problems – Nottingham University Press

INDEX

Ad-lib hopper, 15
Aerial contaminants, 38
Air changes, 37
Air inlet, 10, 61, 68
Air movement, 19
Air quality, 38
Air temperature, 1
Alarm trigger point, 69
Alarm unit, 25, 59, 60, 69
All-in/all- out, 10
Ambient temperature, 38, 61, 62, 70, 71
Ammonia, 29, 37, 38
Auger, 15, 16, 45, 52
Automatic control of natural ventilation
    (ACNV), 20, 21, 22

Barn report, 6, 51, 53
Body clock, 43
Body heat, 59
British Pig Executive Yearbook, 75
Broadband, 5, 6, 7
Bulk storage bin, 53

Carbon dioxide, 32
Cellular, 1, 5
Climatic environment, 8, 14
Code of Recommendations of Livestock
    - Pigs, xii, 12
Contract pig finishing, 54
Control equipment, 11
Controlled environment, 1
Creep heating, 27
Creep lamp, 25, 26, 27

Data logger, 2, 4, 5, 6, 16, 17
Data logging, 6, 53
Dicam®, 5
Digital thermometer, 2
Dry fed, 15

Early adopters, 8
Electrical consumption, 18
Embedded intelligence, 78
Environmental monitoring, 15, 24, 29
Evaporative cooling, 69

Fan controller, 31
Fan switch, 39, 40, 41
Fan ventilated, 15
Farrowing rooms, 25, 61, 68
Feed conversion efficiency, 47
Feed costs, 43
Feed delivery, 51, 53, 54, 55
Feed intake, 17, 46, 50
Feed use, 18
Finishing pig building, 15, 22
Five freedoms, 11
Float valve, 56
Food chain, 74

Group size, 14
GPRS, 78
GSM, 78

Header tank, 56
Heat input, 29
Heuristics, 3
Humidity, 18

Information technology (IT), vii, 6, 7, 8,
    9, 10, 14, 75, 76
Internet, 6, 77, 88
Interval timer, 31

Landline modem, 5
Lower critical temperature, 19
Lying behaviour, 38

Maintenance, 46, 48, 49
Maximum/minimum temperature, 27

Maximum/minimum thermometer, xii, 1
Maximum ventilation rate, 35
Minimum ventilation rate, 29, 31, 32, 35, 37, 38
M2M technology, 77, 78

Naturally ventilated building, 19
Noxious gases, 29, 30, 32, 38

Odours, 29
Over-ventilation, 34, 35

Physical environment, 14
Pigmeat consumption, 73
Proportional band, 22

Quality assurance schemes, xii

RCD, 62
Real time monitoring, 3, 4
RS485 network, 4

Satellite, 6
Sensor, 4
Set temperature, 70
SIM card, 77
Slatter floor, 57
Solar gain, 24
Space allowance, 11, 13
Speed control, 31
Stocking density, 10
Stocking rate, 13

Temperature control, 19, 25
Temperature differential, 36
Temperature fluctuation, 20, 23, 36,
Temperature gradient, 24
Temperature lift, 60, 69, 70
Temperature target, 38
Temperature variation, 19, 18, 37
Time to trigger, 64, 67

Upper critical temperature, 19

Ventilation capacity, 37
Ventilation failure, 65, 66
Ventilation flaps, 20
Ventilation rates, 29, 31, 32, 33
Water, 47, 54, 58
Water consumption, 54
Water flow, 18, 56, 57
Water intake, 16, 44, 45
Water logging trace, 56
Water meter, 15, 16
Water storage, 44
Water supply, 46, 55
Welfare, xii, 11
Welfare of Farm Animals (England) (Amendments) Regulations 2003, xii
WiFi, 67
Wind effect, 24
Wind speeds, 24, 38
Wireless connectivity, 79
Wireless (radio), 6
Wireless technology, 4